CONTENTS

Chapter One: Sex Matters

Chapter Two: Improving Sexual Health

Useful information for readers

Dear Reader,

Issues: Sexual Health

Myths and misinformation about sexual matters are all too prevalent, especially among young people. ChildLine receives nearly 50 calls a day about sex, and the total number of diagnosed sexually transmitted infections in those aged 16 to 19 rose by 24% between 2003 and 2007. This title covers sexual relationships, risky sexual behaviour, the rise of STIs and the ways in which these can be prevented and treated. It also covers the debate surrounding the provision of sex education in schools.

The purpose of *Issues*

Sexual Health is the one hundred and seventy-third volume in the **Issues** series. The aim of this series is to offer up-to-date information about important issues in our world. Whether you are a regular reader or new to the series, we do hope you find this book a useful overview of the many and complex issues involved in the topic. This title replaces an older volume in the **Issues** series, Volume 96: **Preventing Sexual Diseases,** which is now out of print.

Titles in the **Issues** series are resource books designed to be of especial use to those undertaking project work or requiring an overview of facts, opinions and information on a particular subject, particularly as a prelude to undertaking their own research.

The information in this book is not from a single author, publication or organisation; the value of this unique series lies in the fact that it presents information from a wide variety of sources, including:
⇨ Government reports and statistics
⇨ Newspaper articles and features
⇨ Information from think-tanks and policy institutes
⇨ Magazine features and surveys
⇨ Website material
⇨ Literature from lobby groups and charitable organisations.*

Critical evaluation

Because the information reprinted here is from a number of different sources, readers should bear in mind the origin of the text and whether the source is likely to have a particular bias or agenda when presenting information (just as they would if undertaking their own research). It is hoped that, as you read about the many aspects of the issues explored in this book, you will critically evaluate the information presented. It is important that you decide whether you are being presented with facts or opinions. Does the writer give a biased or an unbiased report? If an opinion is being expressed, do you agree with the writer?

Sexual Health offers a useful starting point for those who need convenient access to information about the many issues involved. However, it is only a starting point. Following each article is a URL to the relevant organisation's website, which you may wish to visit for further information.

Kind regards,

Lisa Firth
Editor, **Issues** series

* Please note that Independence Publishers has no political affiliations or opinions on the topics covered in the Issues series, and any views quoted in this book are not necessarily those of the publisher or its staff.

ISSUES TODAY
A RESOURCE FOR KEY STAGE 3

Younger readers can also now benefit from the thorough editorial process which characterises the **Issues** series with the launch of a new range of titles for 11- to 14-year-old students, **Issues Today**. In addition to containing information from a wide range of sources, rewritten with this age group in mind, **Issues Today** titles also feature comprehensive glossaries, an accessible and attractive layout and handy tasks and assignments which can be used in class, for homework or as a revision aid. In addition, these titles are fully photocopiable. For more information, please visit the **Issues Today** section of our website (www.independence. co.uk).

Sex

Sex is normal in loving relationships between couples above the age of consent. It's not compulsory in any relationship, but you owe it to yourself to find out as much as you can about sex and how to keep yourself safe before making any decisions

It can be really difficult to talk about sex and contraception, as it's a private and personal thing. You might feel like you'll be judged if you are having sex, or if you're not, or feel silly if you have questions. Everyone has questions or worries about sex and it's normal to feel like this.

If you are thinking about having sex, it's best to find out about it and take responsibility for what you are doing. It's a good idea to discuss things with the person you are going to have sex with, so that you both know what you are doing.

Is it normal to have lots of questions about sex?

It's completely normal to have lots of questions about sex, both before or after you have sex. You should be able to ask whatever you want and not be embarrassed. The more you know the fewer risks you're likely to take, as it is important to keep yourself safe if or when you enter into a sexual relationship.

At what age can I have sex?

In the UK, you can legally have sex after the age of 16 (from 2 February 2009 the law in Northern Ireland changed from 17 years old to 16 years old). This applies to heterosexual sex (between a male and female), or homosexual or gay sex (between two members of the same sex). Although you can legally have sex at these ages, you should only have sex when you are ready and not feel pressured into doing it.

I'm having lots of sexual thoughts and feelings, is this normal?

It's normal to have sexual thoughts and feelings, especially during puberty when your body is changing. It can be confusing and strange at first but it isn't unusual. Your feelings should calm down after a while when your body adjusts to the changes.

I'm worried about having sex, am I weird?

It's natural to have worries about having sex, as it's a big step to take. The most important things are that you are happy with what you do and that you are safe.

If you are unsure about it or feel uncomfortable about having sex, then it probably means that it's not the right time for you.

Here are some wrong reasons to have sex:
⇨ You think it'll help you feel grown up.
⇨ Your mates say they've done it and you don't want to be left out.
⇨ You're worried what will happen if you say no.
⇨ Someone is pressuring you into doing it.
⇨ You just want someone to love you.

What is contraception and why should I use it?

Contraception, or birth control, is when you take some action to prevent a pregnancy or sexually transmitted infection (STI). Not everyone knows about contraception. Even when they do, they don't always use it. Even if it is the first time having sex for both of you, you should always use contraception.

Using contraception can help you to:
⇨ Avoid pregnancy when you have sex with someone.
⇨ Avoid STIs such as Chlamydia, gonorrhea, syphilis, and the HIV virus which can lead to AIDS.

There are lots of different types of contraception available and so you'll be able to find one that suits you. You can talk to a doctor or family planning advisor about all your contraceptive options, or visit www.brook.org.uk

If you are worried about anything to do with sex or contraception, you can talk to us about your worries and we can help. We respect children and young people regardless of their age or gender or sexuality, and you can talk to us about any of your worries without being judged.

It's completely normal to have lots of questions about sex

Further advice
⇨ Brook Advisory Centres – commonly known just as Brook – is the only national voluntary sector provider of free and confidential sexual health advice and services specifically for young people under 25. Visit www.brook.org.uk
⇨ likeitis gives young people access to information about all aspects of sex education and teenage life. Visit www.likeitis.org.uk
⇨ ruthinking includes advice about issues related to sex, health and growing up. Visit www.ruthinking.co.uk

⇨ Information from ChildLine. Visit www.childline.org.uk for more.

Copyright © NSPCC – All rights reserved. National Society for the Prevention of Cruelty to Children. ChildLine is a service provided by NSPCC, Weston House, 42 Curtain Road, London EC2A 3NH. In Scotland the ChildLine service is provided by Children 1st on behalf of the NSPCC. Registered charity numbers 216401 and SC037717.

Sex and relationships

Frequently asked questions

My girlfriend/boyfriend wants me to have sex and I think I want to. Should I?

If you're unsure about having sex, it might be worth talking to a counsellor about your feelings. Remember that there are different ways of giving each other pleasure, apart from full sex. It's important not to feel pressurised into doing anything that you're not ready for. If you are thinking of having sex, then it's also important to get advice about contraception to avoid pregnancy and sexually transmitted infections.

I'm 15 years old and all my friends are having sex but I don't feel ready to – am I normal?

Yes! Around 30% of young men and women have had sex before the age of 16, so that means 70% – the majority – haven't. Peer pressure on young people to have sex can be intense, but what's right for one person isn't necessarily right for someone else. And the younger the age at which people first have sex, the more likely they are to say they regret it later.

I'm not ready to sleep with my boyfriend but he says if I loved him I would. What should I do?

It's important not to be pushed into doing something that you're not ready for. It must be your choice to have sex and you have every right to wait until you feel that the time is right. Your boyfriend is using emotional blackmail to get you to do something you don't want. Be honest with him and tell him how you feel. Explain that it doesn't mean that you don't love him, simply that you are not ready for sex. Love is caring about another person. If he loves you, he will respect your decision.

I think that I masturbate too much even though I'm in a relationship. What's normal?

Masturbation is natural and harmless for men and for women. It is a way of exploring your own body and can help you to find out what you like and don't like sexually. It is fine to masturbate as often or little as you like.

My girlfriend's refusing to have sex with me without a condom but I don't like using condoms. What should I do?

If you want to have penetrative sex, where the penis enters the vagina, anus or mouth, it is important to practise safer sex by using a condom to reduce the risk of getting sexually transmitted infections, including HIV, as well as reducing the risk of pregnancy.

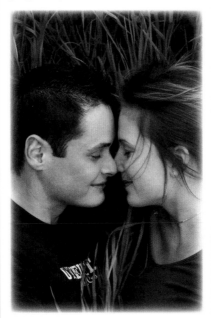

You and your girlfriend may also want to explore other ways of giving each other pleasure involving non-penetrative forms of safer sex where there is no contact between both your bodily fluids (blood, semen, vaginal fluids) such as mutual masturbation.

I had sex with my boyfriend for the first time and I bled. Is this normal?

First time sex can hurt and some women do bleed a little bit if the hymen (a small piece of thin skin which covers some of the opening of the vagina) is still intact, as it will break the first time you have sexual intercourse. This doesn't happen in all women as the hymen may already have broken before sex, e.g. through using tampons.

I've had sex with my boyfriend a few times and it hurts. Do you think something's wrong?

Pain during sex can happen for different reasons. It could be because you are tense, or not aroused enough. Taking things slowly and using extra lubrication, like KY jelly, can help, but if you are tense and worried about sex, you may want to go along to a local service to see a family planning nurse and/or a counsellor. Pain during sex can also be a symptom of a sexually transmitted infection. If you think that you may have a sexually transmitted infection, you should go to a Genito-Urinary Medicine (GUM) clinic for testing and treatment.

I had sex with my girlfriend and climaxed too early. Is there something wrong?

Premature ejaculation is the most common sexual problem affecting men. It happens to most men at some time and there is nothing to worry about. If you're really worried, you can get advice on techniques that can help from your GP or local family planning clinic, or a specialist organisation.

I didn't get an erection during sex. Is there something wrong?

This is a common problem amongst men and can have physical or psychological causes. For example, anxiety can affect erections, as can drinking alcohol before sex. If you're really worried, you can get help and treatment from your GP or local family planning clinic, or a specialist organisation.

⇨ The above information is reprinted with kind permission from Brook. Visit www.brook.org.uk for more information.

© Brook

Sexual health in 2008

Illustrative examples

Sexual behaviour

⇨ 51% of people said they would always, and 14% said they would never or rarely, use a condom with a new sexual partner.[i]

⇨ Of men who had sex with another man over the last year, 36% were consistent condom users. 53% had had anal sex at least once without a condom.[ii]

⇨ Frequent use of alcohol and other drugs is associated with high numbers of sexual partners and decreased likelihood of using protection.[iii]

Contraception

⇨ The most frequently used method is the contraceptive pill (27%) followed by the male condom (22%).[iv]

⇨ Only 10% of women under 50 report using long-acting reversible contraception as their method of contraception although 45% would use this method if offered.[v]

Pregnancy and abortion

⇨ The teenage conception rate declined by 13.3% (in 15-17s) between 1998 and 2006.[vi]

⇨ Abortion rates are highest in 18- to 24-year-olds, peaking at age 19 (36 per 1000 women aged 19, compared to 18 per 1000 aged 15-44).[vii]

⇨ 68% of NHS-funded abortions in 2007 took place at under 10 weeks compared with 51% in 2002 (a 33% increase).[vii]

⇨ The proportion of medical abortions has more than doubled in the last five years, reaching 35% of all abortions in 2007.[vii]

⇨ 32% of all women undergoing abortion in 2007 had had one or more previous procedures (28% of Asian women, 48% of Black women).[v]

Sexually transmitted infections

⇨ Numbers of new STI diagnoses at GUM clinics have risen steadily over the last 10 years. The highest rates are in young people and men who have sex with men (MSM).[viii]

⇨ 16- to 24-year-olds account for nearly half of all STIs diagnosed in GUM clinics.[ix]

⇨ Men who have sex with men account for a fifth of new diagnoses of gonorrhea and over half of new episodes of syphilis seen in GUM.[x]

51% of people said they would always, and 14% said they would never or rarely, use a condom with a new sexual partner

---

⇨ 9.5% of women and 8.4% of men aged under 25 test positive for Chlamydia when screened.[ix]

⇨ Black Caribbeans continue to have a very high incidence of STIs, accounting for 17% of all gonorrhea diagnoses though they only comprise 1% of the UK population.[xi]

HIV[xi]

⇨ 73,000 people are estimated to be living with HIV in the UK, including one-third who are unaware of their diagnosis.

⇨ An estimated 43% of those living with HIV are men who have sex with men, and 35% are people born in sub-Saharan Africa.

⇨ Over 52,000 people accessed care for HIV in 2006, a tripling in numbers since 1997. The increase was greatest in London, but the largest proportionate increases were outside London.

⇨ Late diagnosis accounts for 35% of HIV-related deaths.[xii] An estimated one-third of all HIV diagnoses and 40% of those in black Caribbeans and black Africans occur late (CD4 count <200).

Public knowledge and attitudes

⇨ 79% of people were aware HIV could be passed on by sex between a man and woman without a condom in 2007, 12% less than in 2000.[i]

⇨ 70% believe that people with HIV deserve the same level of support and respect as someone with cancer, compared to 77% in 2000.[i]

⇨ One-third of people living with HIV in London reported being discriminated against because of their infection, almost half of these saying this had involved a healthcare worker.[xiii]

⇨ 40% of young people state that the quality of sex and relationships education in schools is poor or very poor.[xiv]

⇨ 30-50% of people in secondary schools attracted to the opposite sex have directly experienced homophobic bullying.[xv]

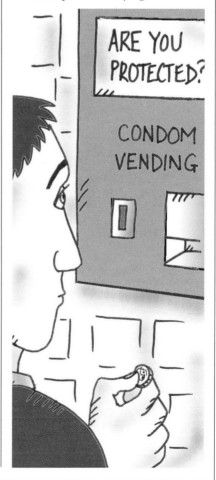

ARE YOU PROTECTED?

CONDOM VENDING

Sources

i National AIDS Trust (2007) *Public attitudes towards HIV.*

ii Weatherburn P, Hickson F, Reid D et al (2008) *Multiple chances: findings from the United Kingdom Gay Men's Sex Survey 2006.* Sigma Research.

iii Bellis M, in *Independent Advisory Group on Sexual Health and HIV report* (2007). 'Sex, drugs, alcohol and young people: a review of the impact drugs and alcohol have on young people's sexual behaviour'.

iv *National Statistics Omnibus Survey* (2007). 'Contraception and Sexual Health 2006/07'. Office for National Statistics.

v Armstrong N, Davey C, Donaldson C (2005) *The economics of sexual health.* fpa.

vi Office for National Statistics and Teenage Pregnancy Unit, 2008.

vii Department of Health (2008) *Abortion statistics, England and Wales: 2007.*

viii HPA (2008) *Continued increase in sexually transmitted infections: an analysis of data from UK genito-urinary medicine clinics up to 2007.*

ix HPA (2008) *Sexually transmitted infections and young people in the United Kingdom: 2008 report.*

x HPA (2008) *All new STI episodes seen at GUM clinics in the UK: 1998-2007.*

xi Health Protection Agency (2007) *Testing times: HIV and other sexually transmitted infections in the UK.*

xii British HIV Association *Clinical Audit Report 2005–6* (2006) 'HIV related deaths in the HAART era'.

xiii Elford J et al (2007) 'HIV-related discrimination reported by people living with HIV in London, UK'. *AIDS and Behavior,* vol 12, no 2, p255-64.

xiv UK Youth Parliament (2007) *Are you getting it?*

xv Hunt R (2007) *Speak Out.* Stonewall.

July 2008

⇨ The above information is an extract from *Progress and priorities – working together for high quality sexual health,* published by the Medical Foundation for AIDS & Sexual Health and reprinted with permission. Visit www.medfash.org.uk for more information.

© Medical Foundation for AIDS & Sexual Health

Sexual experiences of young people aged 14 to 17 – survey

In your opinion which ONE of the following has given you the MOST valuable advice about sex and relationships?

- None of the above – I haven't had any valuable advice about sex – 3%
- Over-18 Internet sites/magazines – 2%
- Other 2%
- Don't know/prefer not to say – 3%
- Teen magazines/books/Internet sites – 10%
- Parents/guardians 34%
- Friends 23%
- School/teachers 23%

To what extent do you agree or disagree with each of the following statements?

- ■ Agree strongly
- ■ Tend to agree
- □ Neither agree nor disagree
- ■ Tend to disagree
- ▨ Disagree strongly
- ▨ Don't know/prefer not to say

Statement	Agree strongly	Tend to agree	Neither agree nor disagree	Tend to disagree	Disagree strongly	Don't know/prefer not to say
I need more information and education about sex and relationships	4	24%	28%	27%	14%	2
I am always honest with friends about my sexual activity	15%	32%	26%	18%	4	5%
Me and my friends frequently talk about sex	16%	41%	23%	13%	5%	2
Sex is discussed openly in my family	11%	30%	24%	19%	15%	
I am always honest with my parents about my sexual activity	13%	22%	22%	20%	15%	7%

At which age did you first have sex (full sexual intercourse)?

Age	%
Under 11	0%
12	0%
13	1%
14	4%
15	8%
16	6%
17	2%
Don't know/prefer not to say/never had sex	78%

We would like you to consider your experience of sexual activity. This includes intercourse, oral sex or mutual masturbation. At which age did you have your first sexual experience?

- Under 11 – 1%
- 12 – 2%
- 13 – 6%
- 14 – 10%
- 15 – 11%
- 16 – 7%
- 17 – 2%
- Don't know/prefer not to say/never had sexual experience 61%

How many sexual partners have you had?

	%
None	64%
One	11%
Two	6%
Three to five	3%
Six to ten	1%
More than ten	1%
Don't know/prefer not to say	15%

Base: 1424 young people aged 14 to 17. Fieldwork: 18-21 July 2008. Source: YouGov (www.yougov.com).

Sex myths

It's amazing what some people believe about sex. Here are some common mistaken ideas

You can't get pregnant during un-protected sex if the man pulls out before he ejaculates (cums) – false!
Even though your boyfriend doesn't ejaculate, sperm can still be present in his pre-cum (the clear, sticky drops that are released when he's aroused). It only takes one sperm to get you pregnant, and the fluid can also contain sexually transmitted infections. Some men aren't aware that they are ejaculating until it's too late, and it's easy to get carried away in the heat of the moment.

You can't get pregnant during your period – false!
There's a chance that you can get pregnant during a period, part-icularly towards the end of your menstrual cycle. Unprotected sex also increases the risk of infection by sexually transmitted infections (STIs).

You can't get pregnant while having sex standing up, or in the shower or bath – false!
If you have unprotected sex you can get pregnant, no matter how or where you do it.

Condoms are 100% safe – false!
Condoms are a highly effective form of contraception, as well as a great way of preventing STIs. However, condoms can and do break, so it's always good to use them in conjunction with another form of contraception such as the pill.

You can't get pregnant while on the pill – false!
The chances of getting pregnant while taking the contraceptive pill are virtually nil, providing you follow the instructions correctly and consistently. But if you miss pills, are on antibiotics, or have sickness and diarrhoea, you need to use condoms for the next seven days.

It's safe to have sex as soon as you're on the pill – false!
Different types of contraceptive pill take different times to kick in. This can range from 0-14 days. Always follow the instructions prescribed with your type of pill, and use an additional form of contraception such as condoms during the time it takes for your choice of pill to become effective.

Missing one pill doesn't matter – false!
The contraceptive pill should be taken at the same time each day, but is regarded as 'missed' if it is taken more than 12 hours late (three hours late for the mini pill, although with the mini pill Cerazette you have a 12-hour window). If you are late in taking your contraceptive, take a pill as soon as you can, then another at the usual time (even if this means taking more than one pill in one day).

If more than one pill is missed, the last missed pill should be taken and the rest of the packet taken at the

normal time. However, alternative contraception (such as condoms) should also be used for seven days afterwards, just to be on the safe side.

If you miss a pill and there are less than seven pills left in the pack, the course should be finished as usual and a new packet started immediately afterwards without a break.

If a condom breaks, there's nothing you can do – false!
If you're female and the condom has split, even if it's before your partner has ejaculated, seek emergency contraception.

The emergency contraceptive pill (morning-after pill) must be started within 72 hours of sex. The IUD (coil) must be fitted within five days after sex. Both are available from your doctor or GUM clinic (contact your local hospital for details). Emergency contraception is not an option to be considered before sex. It is exactly what is says: a last resort should your main form of contraception fail.

Peeing after sex washes out sperm and prevents pregnancy – false!
For a start, urine exits the bladder through the urethra, which lies above the vaginal opening. Which means any sperm in the vagina won't even get wet when you wee.

All guys hate using condoms – false!
The only guys who WON'T use condoms are those with no respect for you. Don't rely on a lad to provide condoms. If you're considering sex then take responsibility for yourself. Get clued up about contraception and safer sex.

⇨ The above information is reprinted with kind permission from TheSite. Visit www.thesite.org for more information.

© TheSite

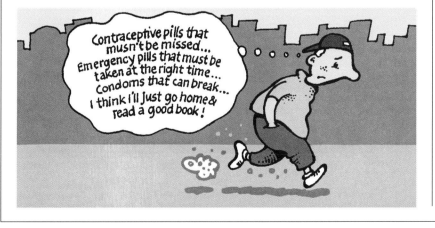

Britain 'most promiscuous Western nation'

Information from Seduction Labs

In an international index measuring one-night stands, total numbers of partners and attitudes towards sex, Britain comes out ahead of America, Australia, France, Germany, Italy and the Netherlands; making the British the most promiscuous of any large western industrial nation.

The study was conducted by asking more than 14,000 people in 48 countries to fill in an anonymous questionnaire about their attitudes towards casual sex and how many people they expected to sleep with over the next five years. The results were then turned into an index of 'sociosexuality', which measured how sexually liberal people are in thought and behaviour.

Most individuals scored between 4 and 65. Finland ranked highest with an average of 51 and Taiwan came lowest with 19. Britain's average score of 40 placed it 11th overall – behind countries such as Latvia, Croatia and Slovenia, but highest amongst major western industrial nations.

The researchers behind the study suggest that high scores might be correlated to the way society is increasingly willing to accept sexual promiscuity among women as well as men. Cultural developments have also meant women are now able to engage in no-strings sex as much as men.

David Schmitt, a Professor of Psychology at Bradley University, Illinois, who oversaw the research, said:

'Historically we have repressed women's short-term mating and there are all sorts of double standards out there where men's short-term mating was sort of acceptable but women's wasn't.'

Britain's high score was attributed to factors such as the decline of religious scruples about extramarital sex, the growth of equal pay and equal rights for women and a highly sexualised popular culture.

Professor Schmitt pointed out that the ratio of men to women is one of the factors that determines a country's ranking, noting that high scores in many Baltic and eastern European states could be linked to the fact that women outnumber men, and thus are under more pressure to conform to what men want in order to find a mate. By contrast, in Asian countries, men tend to slightly outnumber women, so it is the men who have to conform to what women want.

The findings are backed up by earlier research showing that the British are more likely than other nationalities to have 'stolen' another person's partner, and apparently a third of British men are in relationships with women that they have poached from other long-term relationships. Amongst British women, 28% had poached their boyfriend from another relationship, rather than forming a relationship with a single man.

This compares with America, where just 17% of men had 'stolen' another person's girlfriend. In France only 10% of both men and women were poachers, whilst in Germany the figures were 17% for men and 14% for women.

Interestingly, in more liberal countries such as Britain, women might even be becoming more promiscuous than men, since one of the latest theories emerging from evolutionary psychologists such as Professor Schmitt is the idea that when women are at their most fertile, they become even more willing than men to consider one-night stands.

However, there are still key differences in the behaviours of men and women, especially regarding the ages at which they are most sexually liberated. Schmitt found that men tended to have the most sexual partners, and to try hardest to acquire new ones whilst in their twenties. On the other hand, women's promiscuity and lustful thoughts tended to peak whilst in their thirties.

30 November 2008

⇨ The above information is reprinted with kind permission from Seduction Labs. Visit www.seductionlabs.org for more information.

© Seduction Labs

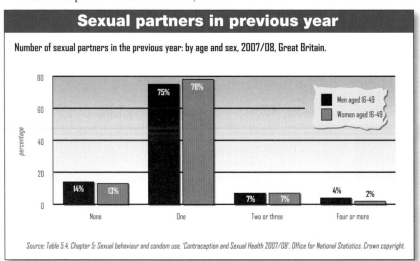

Sexual partners in previous year

Number of sexual partners in the previous year: by age and sex, 2007/08, Great Britain.

Men aged 16-49
Women aged 16-49

None: 14% / 13%
One: 75% / 78%
Two or three: 7% / 7%
Four or more: 4% / 2%

Source: Table 5.4, Chapter 5: Sexual behaviour and condom use, 'Contraception and Sexual Health 2007/08', Office for National Statistics. Crown copyright.

Nearly 50 calls a day to ChildLine about sex

Information from the NSPCC

Nearly 50 children a day call ChildLine because they feel under pressure to have sex or lack basic knowledge about sexual health, relationships, pregnancy and puberty, new figures show today (5 May 2008).

Children as young as 12 call to talk to a counsellor because they are worried they may be pregnant and lack the facts about safe sex, sexual relationships and peer pressure. Some of these calls come from girls who say they feel pressurised into having sex before they are ready.

The latest figures from ChildLine – a service provided by the NSPCC – reveal a worrying level of pressure to have sex and a profound lack of sexual and relationship awareness among young people. A breakdown of statistics shows that boys are just as concerned as girls. Of 11,128 callers about puberty almost half (5,340) came from boys. A further 6,488 young people called to talk about pregnancy.

One 16-year-old boy told ChildLine he had had unprotected sex with a girl for a dare and was now concerned he might have caught a disease. A 14-year-old girl said that her boyfriend wanted to have sex with her but she did not know how to do it. Another young girl rang to say she was worried she was pregnant after she didn't dare to say 'no' to sex with her boyfriend in case he dumped her.

Head of ChildLine Sue Minto said: 'Children are in the dark about the biological and emotional aspects of sex. This leaves them without the knowledge and skills they need to make informed, responsible decisions about their actions, and so they are getting caught up in sexual situations that could have serious implications in their lives.'

The release of the new figures coincides with a government re-view looking at the way Sex and Relationships Education is taught in schools in England. As part of this review, the NSPCC – a member of the Sex Education Forum – is calling for Personal, Social, Health and Economic Education (PSHE), which includes Sex and Relationships Education, to be made a compulsory part of the school curriculum in England and to be delivered by staff with specialist training.

Children as young as 12 call to talk to a counsellor because they are worried they may be pregnant

---

As the law stands, schools in England only have to teach the biological aspects of sex rather than discuss topics like emotions and relationships, what it means to be pressurised into having sex, and the consequences of risky behaviour. All of these topics form the cornerstone of PSHE.

Sue Minto continued: 'Keeping children safe means giving them the appropriate facts about sex and emotions. This includes discussing peer pressure, relationships and love, and helping young people develop the skills and confidence to make the right decisions for them about sex and keep themselves safe from those who may want to abuse or exploit them.

'Parents also have a responsibility to talk to their children about sex and relationships. But they too need advice and support so they can tackle the subject in a confident and knowledgeable way.

'Children and young people must be armed with the knowledge they need to keep themselves safe. We must not shy away from talking to them honestly and openly about the basic facts. PSHE should not be seen as an optional extra. Nor should it be the missing page in a young person's school textbook.'
5 May 2008

⇨ Information from ChildLine. Visit www.childline.org.uk for more.

Copyright © NSPCC – All rights reserved. National Society for the Prevention of Cruelty to Children. ChildLine is a service provided by NSPCC, Weston House, 42 Curtain Road, London EC2A 3NH. In Scotland the ChildLine service is provided by Children 1st on behalf of the NSPCC. Registered charity numbers 216401 and SC037717.

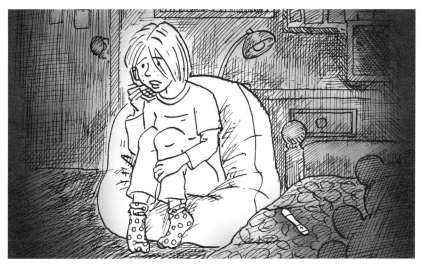

Teenagers: sexual health and behaviour

Information from the fpa

This article aims to provide key data about the sexual health and behaviour of teenagers throughout the United Kingdom (UK). Where possible, data is presented separately for England, Wales, Scotland and Northern Ireland. Please note that this data is not always directly comparable due to differences in methods of data collection and analysis between countries.

Where Great Britain is referred to, this covers England, Wales and Scotland.

Age of consent

⇨ In England, Wales and Northern Ireland, the age of consent to any form of sexual activity is 16 for both men and women, whether they are heterosexual, homosexual or bisexual.[1,2]

⇨ In Scotland, the age of heterosexual consent for women and for sex between men is 16.[3]

⇨ In Scotland, there are no specific laws covering sex between women, so provided both women consent and are 16 or over, this is legal.

Sexual behaviour

The second *National Survey of Sexual Attitudes and Lifestyles* (Natsal 2000), which included over 11,000 men and women aged 16-44 in Great Britain,[4] found that:

⇨ the average (median) age at first heterosexual intercourse was 16 for both men and women;

⇨ nearly a third of men and a quarter of women aged 16–19 had heterosexual intercourse before they were 16;

⇨ about 80 per cent of young people aged 16-24 said that they had used a condom when they first had sex

⇨ less than one in ten had used no contraception at all when they first had sex;

⇨ one in five young men and nearly half of young women aged 16-24 said they wished they had waited longer to start having sex. They were twice as likely to say this if they had been under 15 when they first had sex;

⇨ both young men and women aged 16-24 had had an average of three heterosexual partners in their lifetime[4]

⇨ about one per cent (0.9 per cent men, 1.6 per cent women) of 16- to 24-year-olds had had one or more new same-sex partners in the previous year.[5]

Natsal 2000 did not include Northern Ireland. A separate survey carried out in 2000 by fpa in Northern Ireland and the University of Ulster included over 1,000 young people aged 14-25.[6] It found that:

⇨ the average (median) age at first heterosexual intercourse was 15.6 years (14.9 for men and 15.9 for women);

⇨ just over a third had experienced sexual intercourse before 17 (the legal age of consent in Northern Ireland) and a quarter had sex before 16;

⇨ nearly two-thirds (63.8 per cent) had used a condom when they first had sex, either alone or with another method of contraception;

⇨ about a quarter had used no contraception at all when they first had sex;

⇨ just under a third (31.6 per cent) said they felt they had sex too early, and this was more likely (43 per cent) if they had been under 16 at the time;

⇨ on average, the sexually active 14- to 25-year-olds had had six sexual partners; the average for young women was five, and young men eight.

The sixth annual Gay Men's Sex Survey in 2002[7] included over 16,000 gay and other homosexually active men in the UK aged between 14-83.

⇨ The average age at which men first had any sexual experience with another man was 17.5 years.

⇨ Of those who had engaged in anal intercourse (AI), the average age for first doing so was 20.6 years and 60 per cent had used a condom.

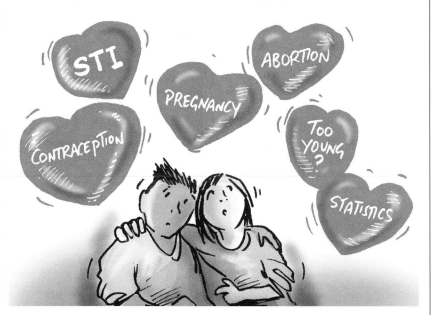

- The first AI partner was, on average, about four years older.
- Men under 20 were significantly more likely to have had both male and female partners (11.3 per cent) than men in other age groups (6.4 per cent-7.9 per cent). In a separate survey of lesbian and bisexual women,[8] the under-20s were more likely to have had sex with both men and women (24 per cent).

The Gay Men's Sex Survey in 2006 found that 25 per cent of men aged 14-19 had had one male sexual partner in the last year, 41 per cent had had two to four, and 34 per cent had had five or more.[9]

Use of contraception

An Office for National Statistics (ONS) survey[10] of women aged 16-49 in Great Britain found that among 16-19 year olds in 2007-08:
- 56 per cent said they used contraception;
- among these, almost equal numbers said they used the pill or condoms (some will use both);
- 86 per cent had heard of emergency hormonal contraception (EHC);
- 7 per cent had used EHC and 1 per cent the emergency IUD at least once in the previous 12 months.

There is no equivalent survey data on contraceptive usage by teenagers in Northern Ireland. The following statistics relate only to women attending community family planning clinics in 2003-04[1.1]
- 49 per cent of women aged 16-19 were using the pill and 21 per cent the condom as their main method of contraception.
- Although women under 20 accounted for 31 per cent of all EC provided through family planning clinics in Northern Ireland, only four per cent of the overall total was those aged under 16.

Use of contraceptive clinic services
- 78,000 women aged under 16 attended family planning clinics in England in 2006-07. This represented 8.3 per cent of the resident population, a slight decrease from 2006-07.[12]
- 255,000 or 19.6 per cent of the resident female population in England aged 16-19 years of age visited a family planning clinic in 2007-08, a slight decrease from 2006-07.[12]

Teenage pregnancy

The UK has the highest teenage birth and abortion rates in Western Europe.[13]

England[14]

In 2006, there were:
- 39,003 under-18 conceptions, a rate of 40.4 per 1,000 females aged 15-17. Nearly half (49 per cent) of the pregnancies were terminated;
- 7,296 under-16 conceptions, a rate of 7.7 per 1,000 females aged 13-15. Over half (60 per cent) of the pregnancies were terminated.

78,000 women aged under 16 attended family planning clinics in England in 2006-07. This represented 8.3 per cent of the resident population

---

Wales[15]

In 2006, there were:
- 2,598 under-18 conceptions, a rate of 44.9 per 1,000 females aged 15-17. Over a third (42.6 per cent) of the pregnancies were terminated;
- 496 under-16 conceptions, a rate of 8.6 per 1,000 females aged 13-15. Over half (53 per cent) of the pregnancies were terminated.

Scotland[16]

(Unlike England and Wales, Scottish conception data includes miscarriages managed in hospitals as well as registered births and abortions.)

In 2006, there were:
- 3,910 under-18 conceptions, a rate of 41.5 per 1,000 females aged 15-17. About 45 per cent of the pregnancies ended in abortion.
- 772 under-16 conceptions, a rate of 8.1 per 1,000 13-15-year-olds. Over half (59 per cent) of the pregnancies ended in abortion.

Northern Ireland

Conception data is not available for Northern Ireland, due to the lack of complete data on the number of women having abortions. Abortion is only legal in Northern Ireland in exceptional circumstances.
- In 2007, 235 teenagers travelled to England to have an abortion,[17] although this number is likely to be an underestimate.
- In 2006, there were 1,427 teenage births (under 20), a rate of 22.5 per 1,000 females aged 15-19.[18]

Abortion

England and Wales[17]
- In 2007, 20,289 women aged under 18 had an abortion. Of these, 4,376 were under 16.
- The under-18 abortion rate was 20.0 per 1,000 and the under-16 rate was 4.0.

Scotland[19]
- In 2007, 3,176 women aged 16-19 and 372 under-16s had an abortion.
- The abortion rate in 16- to 19-year-olds was 24.5 per 1,000.

Northern Ireland (see Teenage pregnancy section)

Sexually transmitted infections[20]
- The total number of new episodes of selected STIs in men and women aged 16-19 years seen at genitourinary medicine (GUM) clinics in the UK rose from 46,856 in 2003 to 58,133 in 2007, an increase of 24 per cent.
- In 2007, the highest rates of diagnoses among young people aged 16-19 were for Chlamydia, genital warts and genital herpes. Rates were higher among women than men in this age group.
- Rates of diagnoses among women aged 16-19 were: Chlamydia (1,423 per 100,000), genital warts (830 per 100,000), genital herpes (210 per 100,000), and gonorrhea (137 per 100,000).
- Rates of diagnoses among men aged 16-19 were Chlamydia (607 per 100,000), genital warts (322 per 100,000), gonorrhea (106 per 100,000) and genital herpes (44 per 100,000).
- Results from the National

Chlamydia Screening Programme in England[21] in 2006-07 showed that around one in ten men and women aged 16-19 tested positive for Chlamydia during the first four years of the programme.

Knowledge of STIs

In an Office for National Statistics survey of around 1,200 adults in Great Britain:[10]

⇨ 87 per cent of men and 94 per cent of women aged 16-24 years knew that Chlamydia is an STI.

Of those respondents who recognised Chlamydia as an STI:

⇨ 66 per cent of men and 73 per cent of women aged 16-24 years old knew that it doesn't always cause symptoms

⇨ 44 per cent of men and 62 per cent of women aged 16-24 years old knew that it is easily treated by antibiotics.

An annual survey of school-aged children shows an apparent decline in anxiety about HIV and AIDS. In 1993, 27 per cent of males and 34 per cent of females aged 14-15 years said that they worried a lot or quite a lot about HIV and AIDS, compared with six per cent and eight per cent in 2003.[22]

References

1 Sexual Offences Act 2003.
2 Sexual Offences (Northern Ireland) Order 2008.
3 Sexual Offences (Scotland) Act 1976; Sexual Offences Amendment Act 2000.
4 Wellings K et al, 'Sexual behaviour in Britain: early heterosexual experience' *Lancet*, vol 358 (2001), 1843–1850.
5 Johnson A et al, 'Sexual behaviour in Britain: partnerships, practices and HIV risk behaviours' *Lancet*, vol 358 (2001), 1835–1842.
6 Schubotz D et al, *Towards Better Sexual Health: A survey of sexual attitudes and lifestyles of young people in Northern Ireland*. Research report (London: fpa, 2003).
7 Hickson F et al, *Out and About. Findings from the United Kingdom Gay Men's Sex Survey 2002* (London: Sigma Research, 2003).

The average (median) age at first heterosexual intercourse was 16 for both men and women

---

8 Henderson L et al, First, Service. *Relationships, sex and health among lesbian and bisexual women* (London: Sigma Research, 2003).
9 Weatherburn T et al, *Multiple Chances: Findings from the United Kingdom Gay Men's Sex Survey 2006* (London: Sigma Research, 2008).
10 Lader D and Hopkins G, *Contraception and Sexual Health, 2007/08* (London: Office for National Statistics, 2008).
11 fpa, *Family Planning Services in Northern Ireland* (Belfast: fpa, 2005).
12 Information Centre, NHS contraceptive services, England: 2007-08 (London: IC, 2008).
13 UNICEF, 'A League Table of Teenage Births in Rich Nations' (Florence: Innocenti Research Centre, 2001).
14 Teenage Pregnancy Unit, *Teenage Conception Statistics for England 1998-2006*.
15 Welsh Assembly Government, Statistical Directorate, *Teenage Conceptions in Wales*, 2006.
16 ISD Scotland, *Teenage Pregnancy Statistics, year ending December 2006*.
17 Department of Health, *Abortion Statistics, England and Wales: 2007* (London: DH, 2008). Statistical Bulletin 2008/01.
18 Northern Ireland Statistics and Research Agency, 'Births', accessed 19 Nov 2008.
19 ISD Scotland, *Abortion*.
20 Health Protection Agency, *Selected STI Diagnoses and Diagnosis Rates from GUM Clinics: 2003–2007* (London: HPA, 2008).
21 National Chlamydia Screening Programme, *Maintaining Momentum. Annual Report of the National Chlamydia Screening Programme, 2006/7* (London, Health Protection Agency, 2007).
22 Schools Health Education Unit, *Trends: Young People – Emotional Health and Well-Being* (Exeter: Schools Health Education Unit, 2004).

February 2009

⇨ The above information is reprinted with kind permission from the **fpa**. Visit www.fpa.org.uk for more information on this and other related topics.

© *fpa*

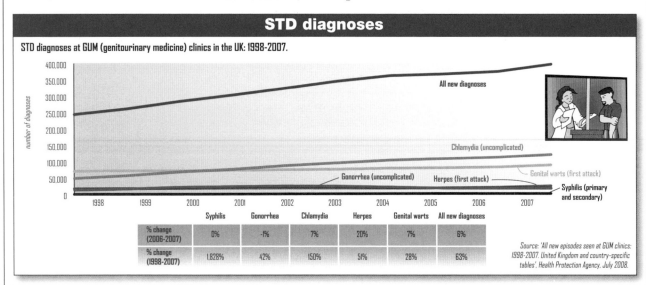

STD diagnoses

STD diagnoses at GUM (genitourinary medicine) clinics in the UK: 1998-2007.

All new diagnoses

Chlamydia (uncomplicated)

Gonorrhea (uncomplicated)   Herpes (first attack)   Genital warts (first attack)

Syphilis (primary and secondary)

	Syphilis	Gonorrhea	Chlamydia	Herpes	Genital warts	All new diagnoses
% change (2006-2007)	0%	-1%	7%	20%	7%	6%
% change (1998-2007)	1,828%	42%	150%	51%	28%	63%

Source: 'All new episodes seen at GUM clinics: 1998-2007. United Kingdom and country-specific tables', Health Protection Agency, July 2008.

Teens, sex and the law

AVERT

Information from AVERT

It seems to many teens that adults are always making a big deal about people having sex under the age of consent. Many young people think that if they feel ready to have sex and they use protection, it is nothing to do with anyone else. But every teen needs to know the laws and what they mean.

Age of consent laws are there to stop young people from being exploited by adults

---

So what does the age of consent mean?

The age of consent is the age when the law says you can agree to have sex. In most countries, until you reach this age you can't legally have sex with anyone, however old they are. Sometimes the law is slightly different when the partners are of a similar age, but there is usually still a minimum age below which sex is always illegal.

But our parents say it's okay. . .

That doesn't make any difference – your parents don't make the law. Teens can't get around the laws for smoking, drinking or driving because their parents say so, and it's the same with this. The age of consent laws always apply, whether you're in love, or you've been together for ages, or you've had sex before.

But it's no-one else's business. Why do we have these laws?

Although many young people are mature enough to know how to deal with it if someone tries to get them to have sex, some teens are not grown up enough to know what to do. Age of consent laws are there to stop young people from being exploited by adults.

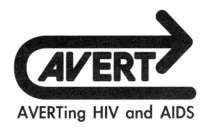

AVERTing HIV and AIDS

What is the age of consent?

What the age of consent is depends on where you live – there are different age limits in different places, and in some places the age of consent is different for boys and for girls. In the UK, the age of consent for both boys and girls is 16 years old.

Is there an age of consent for gay men and lesbians?

Yes. Some places have different age of consent limits for gay men and lesbians, and in other places this sort of relationship is against the law. In the UK, tha age of consent for gay, lesbian and bisexual people is 16 years old.

What is 'statutory rape'?

If you are under the age of consent and you choose to have sex with someone who is over the age of consent, then they can be charged with the crime of 'statutory rape'. Some countries have different names for this crime, and some states in the US call it 'unlawful sexual penetration' or just 'rape'.

And what's sexual abuse?

This is when a person is pressured into any type of sexual contact that they do not agree to. If you know anyone who is being pressurised in this way, you should tell an adult that you trust what's going on. Telephone helplines in your country should also be able to give you advice and information about what you should do and who you should contact. Try the help and advice page on the AVERT website for some suggested resources.

⇨ The above information is reprinted with kind permission from AVERT. Visit www.avert.org for more.
© AVERT

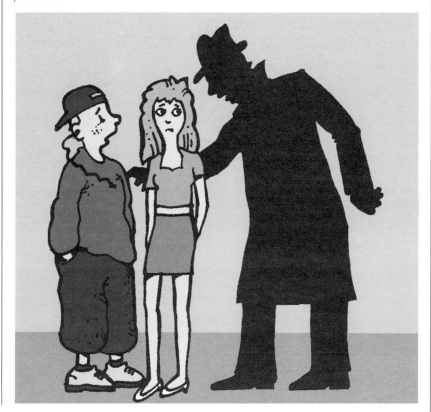

Teens positive about first sexual experience

Young women more likely than young men to report having felt pressure or regret

Most sexually experienced British teens have positive feelings about their first and most recent sexual experiences, according to 'The Quality of Young People's Heterosexual Relationships: A Longitudinal Analysis of Characteristics Shaping Subjective Experience,' by Daniel Wight et al., published in the December 2008 issue of *Perspectives on Sexual and Reproductive Health*. However, a substantial proportion of teens surveyed in Scotland and England (30%) regretted their first intercourse. The proportion who had felt pressured at first sex was roughly twice as high among females as among males (19% vs. 10%), as were the proportions who regretted their first time (38% vs. 20%) and who did not enjoy their most recent sexual experience (12% vs. 5%).

> **The proportion who had felt pressured at first sex was roughly twice as high among females as among males (19% vs. 10%)**

The authors analysed data from two school-based longitudinal studies of 13- to 16-year-olds, and found that of the 42% of youth who reported having had sex by the time of the follow up survey, most assessed their first and most recent sexual relationships positively. Most (81%) also reported feeling no pressure at first intercourse. Those most likely to report feeling pressure from a partner at first sex were female, members of 'other' racial or ethnic groups, and adolescents reporting

poor communication with parents or regular drug use. Additionally, those who had engaged in sex at age 13 or younger were more likely to feel regret than were those who had been 15 to 16 years old, and teens who had first had sex with a boyfriend or girlfriend of more than one month were less likely to feel regret than were those who had first had sex with a casual partner.

The authors suggest that encouraging teens to delay first sex and to restrict sexual activity to close, established relationships can help improve their satisfaction with sexual activity and reduce the number of teens who feel regret about their experiences. They recommend additional research to identify educational or programmatic approaches to develop teens' partner negotiation and communication skills as tools to help them delay premature sexual intercourse, improve their control of sexual encounters and maintain long-term relationships.

9 December 2008

⇨ Source: Guttmacher Institute, *Most British Teens Have Positive Views About Their First Sexual Experience*, news release, New York: Guttmacher, 2008, http://www.guttmacher.org/media/nr/2008/12/09/index.html, accessed 25 March 2009.

© *Guttmacher Institute*

First sexual experience

A survey among 14- to 17-year-olds asked: 'Have you ever had sex? By sex we mean full sexual intercourse.' Results by age of respondent.

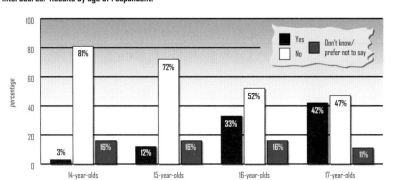

Respondents were also asked: 'At which age did you first have sex? By sex we mean full sexual intercourse.' Results by gender.

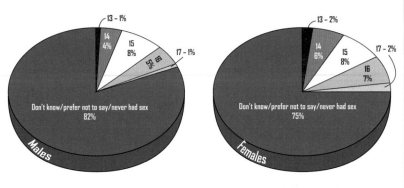

Base: 1424 young people aged 14 to 17. Fieldwork: 18-21 July 2008. Source: YouGov (www.yougov.com).

Under pressure

Boys think it is fine to pressure girls into sex

Teenage boys think there is nothing wrong with using alcohol and other tactics to pressure girls into having sex, a new study has found.

Researchers from Sheffield University presented 14- to 16-year-old boys and girls with different scenarios.

In a situation where a girl was reluctant to have sex with her boyfriend, one boy suggested he could rape her if she continued to resist.

'It became clear that the participants were quite serious – seeming to try to differentiate between "just a bit of pressure" and "proper rape",' the researchers said.

The academics also interviewed girls, but found their responses to be more 'sympathetic'.

'There were no instances where young females used violent or conquest-type language – yet this littered the male responses,' they said.

'This was particularly evident with the alarming manner in which rape was mentioned in two focus groups (with no evidence of disapproval from the other group participants) and also where young men discussed pressurising girls into sex.'

Some of the boys said that 'using tactics like getting a girl drunk were acceptable'.

They recommended that boys need to be involved in 'clear discussion about issues of consent and the withdrawal of consent within sexual encounters'.

The findings will bolster arguments against watering down the age of consent, which some view as a draconian measure that criminalises young people.

But the Home Office has said that adolescents under 18 commit a third of all sex offences, with many of their victims aged 16 or under.

Earlier this year, the Scottish Law Commission and the Children's Commissioner in Scotland proposed that sex between 13- to 15-year-olds should not be an offence under the age of consent law.

MSPs rejected the suggestion, but are now considering whether or not the law should be watered down so that some sexual activity between 13- to 15-year-olds is permitted.

The Christian Institute warns that undermining the age of consent would strip young people of the important protections the law provides.

⇨ The above information is reprinted with kind permission from the Christian Institute. Visit www.christian.org.uk for more.
© Christian Institute

One young person in three has had one-night stand

YouthNet launches *Sex Factor* report

As many as one in three 16- to 24-year-olds (32%) has had a drunken one-night stand they went on to regret, indicates a new report launched on Monday (23 February) by young people's charity, YouthNet.

The *Sex Factor* report presents the attitudes towards sex and sexual health of more than 2,000 16- to 24-year-olds and found that a high proportion had taken part in potentially dangerous sexual activity when drunk.

A third (32%) of young people surveyed said they had had unprotected sex whilst under the influence of alcohol, one in five (22%) said that they had gone home with a 'stranger' and over one in ten (15%) said that they had invited a stranger home with them.

Many young people also expressed disappointment at their 'first time' with one in three sexually active 16- to 24-year-olds (28%) saying that they were unhappy about how they lost their virginity. Choosing the wrong person (75%), being too young (40%) and being in the wrong place (40%) were the top three reasons cited for this unhappiness in the survey.

Almost all of the 16- to 24-year-olds surveyed were sexually active (92%) and more than a third (37%) of those

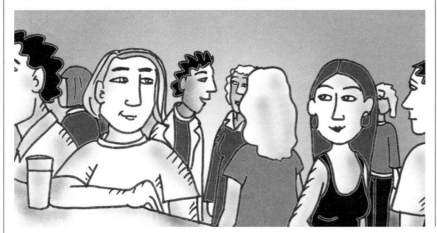

said that they had first had sex under the legal age of 16. Of these, 3% were aged 12 or younger.

TheSite.org relationship expert, Matt Whyman, says: 'Alcohol lowers inhibitions whatever your age, but drink combined with little or no sexual experience can mean dramatic disappointment and regret for young people, or more serious consequences like unplanned pregnancy, STIs or even sexual abuse.

'It's really important that young people take the time to learn about the reality of sex when they're sober, to help them get a real idea of what the risks are, and take steps to make sex safer.'

More than half (55%) of young people who completed the survey agreed that they worried about contracting an STI, and those who had sought advice and information were most likely to use the Internet to search for it, with one in five (22%) respondents saying they had done so in the past.

TheSite.org is the online guide to life for 16- to 24-year-olds and offers advice and guidance on everything from sex and relationships to work and study or drink and drugs.

Young people with questions about sex and relationships – or anything else – can receive a personalised response within three working days at www.thesite.org/askthesite
23 February 2009

⇨ The above information is reprinted with kind permission from YouthNet. Visit www.youthnet.org for more information on this and other related topics.

© *YouthNet*

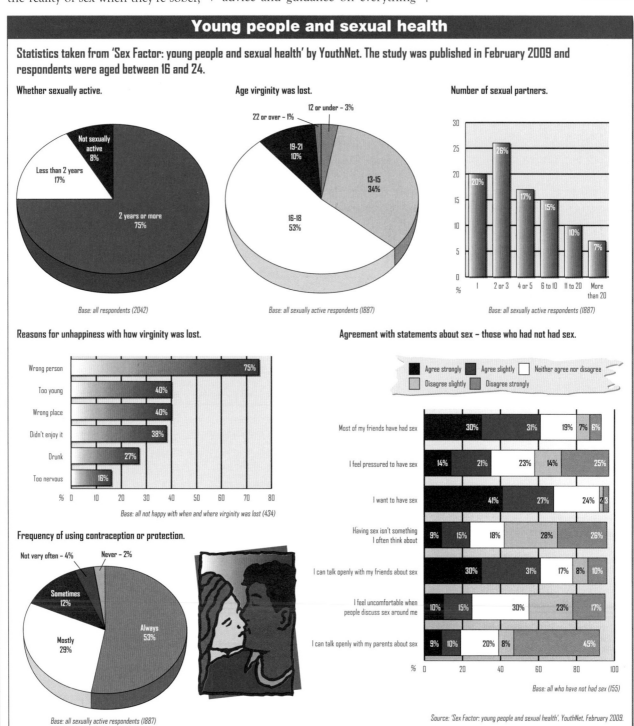

Young people and sexual health

Statistics taken from 'Sex Factor: young people and sexual health' by YouthNet. The study was published in February 2009 and respondents were aged between 16 and 24.

Whether sexually active.
- Not sexually active 8%
- Less than 2 years 17%
- 2 years or more 75%

Base: all respondents (2042)

Age virginity was lost.
- 22 or over – 1%
- 12 or under – 3%
- 19-21 10%
- 13-15 34%
- 16-18 53%

Base: all sexually active respondents (1887)

Number of sexual partners.
- 1: 20%
- 2 or 3: 26%
- 4 or 5: 17%
- 6 to 10: 15%
- 11 to 20: 10%
- More than 20: 7%

Base: all sexually active respondents (1887)

Reasons for unhappiness with how virginity was lost.
- Wrong person 75%
- Too young 40%
- Wrong place 40%
- Didn't enjoy it 38%
- Drunk 27%
- Too nervous 16%

Base: all not happy with when and where virginity was lost (434)

Frequency of using contraception or protection.
- Not very often – 4%
- Never – 2%
- Sometimes 12%
- Mostly 29%
- Always 53%

Base: all sexually active respondents (1887)

Agreement with statements about sex – those who had not had sex.

Legend: Agree strongly | Agree slightly | Neither agree nor disagree | Disagree slightly | Disagree strongly

Statement	Agree strongly	Agree slightly	Neither agree nor disagree	Disagree slightly	Disagree strongly
Most of my friends have had sex	30%	31%	19%	7%	6%
I feel pressured to have sex	14%	21%	23%	14%	25%
I want to have sex	41%	27%	24%	2	3
Having sex isn't something I often think about	9%	15%	18%	28%	26%
I can talk openly with my friends about sex	30%	31%	17%	8%	10%
I feel uncomfortable when people discuss sex around me	10%	15%	30%	23%	17%
I can talk openly with my parents about sex	9%	10%	20%	8%	45%

Base: all who have not had sex (155)

Source: 'Sex Factor: young people and sexual health', YouthNet, February 2009.

Sex and substance abuse

Young people are intentionally taking drink and drugs for better sex

Teenagers and young adults across Europe drink and take drugs as part of deliberate sexual strategies. Findings published in BioMed Central's open access journal, *BMC Public Health*, reveal that a third of 16- to 35-year-old males and a quarter of females surveyed are drinking alcohol to increase their chances of sex, while cocaine, ecstasy and cannabis are intentionally used to enhance sexual arousal or prolong sex.

A third of 16- to 35-year-old males and a quarter of females surveyed are drinking alcohol to increase their chances of sex

---

The study was conducted by researchers in public health and social sciences from across Europe, including LJMU's Centre for Public Health. More than 1,300 people aged between 16 and 35 and who routinely socialise in nightlife settings completed anonymous questionnaires.

Virtually all of the survey participants had drunk alcohol with most having had their first drink when 14 or 15 years old. Three-quarters of the respondents had tried or used cannabis, while around 30 per cent had at least tried ecstasy or cocaine. Overall, alcohol was most likely to be used to facilitate a sexual encounter, while cocaine and cannabis were more likely to be utilised to enhance sexual sensations and arousal.

Despite these perceived sexual 'benefits', drunkenness and drug use were strongly associated with an increase in risk-taking behaviour and feeling regretful about having sex while under the influence of alcohol or drugs. Thus, participants who had been drunk in the past four weeks were more likely to have had five or more partners, sex without a condom and to have regretted sex after drink or drugs in the past 12 months. Cannabis, cocaine or ecstasy use was linked to similar consequences.

'Trends in recent decades have resulted in recreational drug use and binge drinking becoming routine features of European nightlife,' says lead author and Director of LJMU's Centre for Public Health, Professor Mark Bellis. 'Millions of young Europeans now take drugs and drink in ways which alter their sexual decisions and increase their chances of unsafe sex or sex that is later regretted. Yet despite the negative consequences, we found many are deliberately taking these substances to achieve quite specific sexual effects.'

Individuals were significantly more likely to have had sex under 16 years if they had used alcohol, cannabis, cocaine or ecstasy before that age. Girls in particular were as much as four times as likely to have had sex before the age of 16 if they drank alcohol or used cannabis under 16.
9 May 2008

⇨ The above information is reprinted with kind permission from the Centre for Public Health, Liverpool John Moores University. Visit www.cph.org.uk for more information.
© Centre for Public Health, Liverpool John Moores University

Young people and STIs

Young people carry disproportionate burden of sexually transmitted infections in UK

The Health Protection Agency has reported a 6% increase in the total number of new sexually transmitted infections (STIs) diagnosed in 2007 compared to 2006.

To coincide with the launch of the Agency's fifth Annual Report and Accounts, figures are released today showing that across all age groups almost 400,000 (397,990) new STIs were diagnosed in UK genitourinary medicine (GUM) clinics in 2007 – an increase from 375,843 in 2006.

The greatest burden continues to fall among young people (aged 16 to 24 years), who are disproportionately affected by STIs.

While just one in eight of the population are aged 16 to 24 years old, this age group accounts for around half of all newly diagnosed STIs in the UK – 65% of all Chlamydia (79,557 of 121,986), 55% of all genital warts (49,250 of 89,838) and 50% of gonorrhea (9,410 of 18,710) infections diagnosed in GUM clinics last year.

The Health Protection Agency, in its latest publication on sexually transmitted infections and young people, is advising that:
⇨ all sexually active young people are screened for Chlamydia annually and every time they change their sexual partner. Chlamydia, which can have no symptoms, remains the most common sexually transmitted infection;

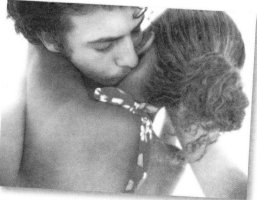

⇨ all gay men should take an HIV test annually and each time they believe themselves to have been at risk of infection;

⇨ people can reduce their risk of catching an STI by having fewer sexual partners and avoiding overlapping sexual relationships;

⇨ everybody should use a condom with a new sexual partner and continue to do so until they have both been screened.

Professor Peter Borriello, Director of the Agency's Centre for Infections, said:

'The number of people being tested for STIs has risen considerably over the past five years, giving us a better insight into the sexual health of the nation. More than one million sexual health screens were carried out in 2007 – a 10% increase on the previous year and one of the reasons why we have seen an increase in the number of diagnoses.

'This increase in testing, together with the decrease we have seen in waiting times for GUM services, ensuring prompt treatment of infections, will help to reduce risk of transmission and the development of complications. If sustained this could have a significant impact on the control of sexually transmitted infections.

'However, we cannot rely on prompt diagnosis and treatment alone – a shift in behaviour is the only way that we will bring down this continued increase in infections.

'Substantial numbers of young people remain undiagnosed, untreated and unaware of the risk they pose both to their own health and that of their sexual partner.

'It is crucial that young people continue to be exposed to messages about safe sex, including condom wearing, and the importance of getting checked out at their nearest GUM clinic if they have had unprotected sex with a new partner.'

New HIV diagnoses in young people remain relatively low compared to older age groups (702 new diagnoses in 2007) although this is still almost three times the number recorded in 1998 (258 diagnoses).

Among young gay men, there has been a substantial increase in the number diagnosed with an STI over the past decade, with more than a doubling of HIV diagnoses between 1998 (128) and 2007 (281) and almost a tripling of gonorrhea diagnoses (339 to 1,001).

___

While just one in eight of the population are aged 16 to 24 years old, this age group accounts for around half of all newly diagnosed STIs in the UK

___

The National Chlamydia Screening Programme in England, which offers sexually active young people screening for Chlamydia and undertakes sexual health activities mainly in the community setting, performed 270,729 screens in 2007 (January to December), a 93% increase on the 140,157 screens performed in 2006. 9.5% of young women and 8.4% of young men tested positive for Chlamydia. This resulted in 24,236 Chlamydia diagnoses in under-25-year-olds.

Justin McCracken, Chief Executive of the Health Protection Agency, said:

'Monitoring of STIs and other infectious diseases forms only one part of the Agency's work in safeguarding the UK's public health. Our fifth annual report illustrates the many other areas in which the Agency has made significant progress in protecting people's health over the last year.

'The Health Protection Agency brings together an exceptionally wide range of skills and experience across the entire public health protection spectrum.

'Firmly embedded at the heart of health protection locally, regionally, nationally and internationally, the Agency is in a unique position to champion public health and help to protect people from radiation, chemical and infectious diseases hazards.

'We are committed to building on the achievements of the first five years of the Agency's development to create an expert body that is widely recognised as authoritative and effective at protecting the health of the public through helping reduce the burden of infectious disease, including sexually transmitted infections.'
15 July 2008

⇨ The above information is reprinted with kind permission from the Health Protection Agency. Visit www.hpa. org.uk for more information.
© *Health Protection Agency*

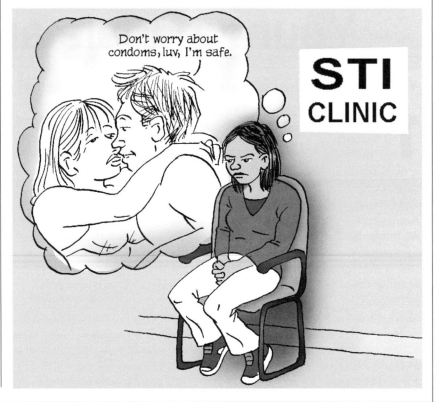

Sexually transmitted diseases and symptoms

Information from AVERT

What are sexually transmitted diseases (STDs)?

Sexually transmitted diseases (STDs) are diseases that are mainly passed from one person to another (that is, transmitted) during sex. There are at least 25 different sexually transmitted diseases with a range of different symptoms. These diseases may be spread through vaginal, anal and oral sex.

Most sexually transmitted diseases will only affect you if you have sexual contact with someone who has an STD. However, there are some infections, for example scabies, which are referred to as STDs because they are most commonly transmitted sexually, but which can also be passed on in other ways.

What are sexually transmitted infections (STIs)?

Sexually Transmitted Infection (STI) is another name for Sexually Transmitted Disease (STD). The name STI is sometimes preferred because there are a few STDs, such as Chlamydia, that can infect a person without causing any actual disease (i.e. unpleasant symptoms). Someone without symptoms may not think of themselves as having a disease, but they may still have an infection that needs treating.

How can you tell if you have a sexually transmitted disease?

You may become aware that you have an STD because of symptoms, or it may be that a sexual partner tells you they have an STD which they might have passed on to you. Some sexually transmitted diseases can be transmitted by an infected person even if they don't have any symptoms.

If you think you might have been exposed to an STD then you should go to see a doctor. Many sexually transmitted diseases can be easily cured, but if left untreated, they may cause unpleasant symptoms and could lead to long-term damage such as infertility. Some STDs can be transmitted from a pregnant woman to her unborn child. It is important that anyone diagnosed with an STD informs everyone they have had sex with within the past year (or everyone following the partner they believe may have infected them).

What are common STD symptoms?

STD symptoms vary, but the most common are soreness, unusual lumps or sores, itching, pain when urinating, and/or an unusual discharge from the genitals.

Which are the most common sexually transmitted diseases?

What follows is a list of some of the most common STDs and other genital diseases. There is also information about HIV transmission and testing and HIV treatment on the AVERT website.

Bacterial Vaginosis (BV) is not strictly an STD as it is not transmitted via sexual intercourse. However, it can be exacerbated by sex and is more frequently found in sexually active women than those who have never had intercourse. It is caused by an imbalance in the normal healthy bacteria found in the vagina and although it is relatively harmless and may pass unnoticed, it can sometimes produce an abundance of unpleasant fishy smelling discharge.

Whilst there is no clear explanation as to why BV occurs, there have been suggestions that the alkaline nature of semen could be one cause, as it may upset the acidic nature of the vaginal bacteria. Another cause can be the use of an intrauterine contraceptive device (coil). A woman cannot pass BV to a man, but it is important she receives treatment as BV can occasionally travel up into the uterus and Fallopian tubes and cause a more serious infection. Treatment for BV consists of applying a cream to the vagina or taking antibiotics.

Chlamydia is one of the most commonly reported bacterial sexually transmitted diseases. It is caused by the Chlamydia trachomatis bacterium. It infects the urethra, rectum and eyes in both sexes, and the cervix in women. If left untreated, long-term infection can lead to fertility problems in women. Chlamydia is transmitted through genital contact and sexual intercourse with someone already infected. Symptoms usually show between 1 and 3 weeks after exposure but may not emerge until much later.

Crabs or Pubic Lice are small crab-shaped parasites that burrow into the skin to feed on blood. They live on coarse body hair, predominantly pubic hair, but can also be found in armpit hair, facial hair and even on eyelashes. The lice are yellow-grey in colour and use their crab-like claws to grip hair strands. They can sometimes be spotted moving on the skin.

Crabs are easily passed on during sex, but can also be passed on through sharing clothes, towels or bedding with someone who has them. Crabs cannot be transmitted via toilet seats or swimming pools.

Crabs symptoms

Symptoms are usually noticed around five days to seven weeks after infection and include:
⇨ itchy skin;
⇨ inflammation of the affected area;
⇨ sometimes visible lice and eggs;
⇨ spots of blood as lice feed from blood vessels in the skin.

Although there is no effective way to prevent becoming infected during sex, a person who has crabs can reduce the risk to others by washing bedding, towels and clothes on a hot wash to kill off the parasites.

Treatment for pubic lice is easy, consisting of special shampoos, lotions and creams that kill off the lice and their eggs. It is not necessary to shave pubic hair as this is unlikely to remove all lice.

Genital warts are caused by some sub-types of human papillomavirus (HPV). They can appear on the skin anywhere in the genital area as small whitish or flesh-coloured bumps, or larger, fleshy, cauliflower-like lumps. They are unlikely to cause pain but may itch and can be difficult to spot. Often there are no other symptoms, but if a woman has a wart on her cervix she may experience slight bleeding or unusual coloured vaginal discharge.

Gonorrhea (once known as the clap) is a sexually transmitted infection that can infect the urethra, cervix, rectum, anus and throat. Symptoms usually appear between 1 and 14 days after exposure, but it is possible to have no symptoms.

Gonorrhea symptoms

Men are more likely to notice symptoms than women. Symptoms can include:

⇨ a burning sensation when urinating;

⇨ a white/yellow discharge from the penis;

⇨ a change in vaginal discharge;

⇨ irritation or discharge from the anus (if the rectum is infected).

Hepatitis is the ancient Greek term for 'liver inflammation'. Hepatitis can occur following excessive and prolonged consumption of alcohol or the use of certain medicines and drugs, but it is most commonly caused by a virus. Several different types of hepatitis virus exist (labelled A to G), with hepatitis A, B and C being the most common. Each viral strain has

different routes of transmission but all damage the liver.

Herpes is caused by two strains of the herpes simplex virus, type 1 (HSV-1) and type 2 (HSV-2). HSV-2 is more common and usually manifests itself in the genital and anal area, whereas HSV-1 is more likely to affect the mouth and lips in the form of cold sores. On a global scale, HSV-2 is a very common STD; for example research suggests that one in five Americans is a carrier of HSV-2. Symptoms of herpes usually appear two to seven days after first exposure to the virus and last two to four weeks.

Herpes symptoms

Both men and women may have multiple symptoms that include:

⇨ itching or tingling sensations in the genital or anal area;

⇨ small fluid-filled blisters that burst, leaving small painful sores;

⇨ pain when passing urine over the open sores (especially in women);

⇨ headaches;

⇨ backache;

⇨ flu-like symptoms, including swollen glands or fever.

Once the first outbreak of blisters has gone, the herpes virus hides away in nerve fibres near the infection site, where it remains dormant, causing no symptoms. Symptoms may come back later (particularly during times of stress and illness) but usually in less severe and shorter episodes.

Molluscum contagiosum (MC, also known as water warts) is a common viral infection resulting in a skin disease that presents itself as small pearl-shaped papules (bumps or lesions), often in clusters. Usually between one to five millimetres in diameter, they are filled with a gungy white fluid that is very contagious. The papules usually appear on exposed skin such as the torso, thighs, genitalia and anus.

They usually develop two to eight weeks after initial infection. MC can be transmitted through direct skin-to-skin contact and also indirectly through sharing towels, baths or clothing with someone infected. It is not strictly an STD as it often occurs in

children, especially those prone to skin conditions such as eczema. Children are more likely to assist transmission by scratching the infected sites, although it should be noted that the chance of passing on the virus is small.

MC is grouped with sexual infections because of the risk of transmission through close body contact during sex, which is why it is often screened for in sexual health clinics.

Reducing MC risks

The risk of becoming infected with MC can be reduced by:

⇨ using condoms during sex, although this only offers partial protection as MC can be passed on by anal/genital lesions not covered by the condom;

⇨ covering affected areas of skin (where possible) with clothing or sterile dressings;

⇨ not sharing baths, clothing and towels.

The recommended treatment is often to leave MC to clear up by itself (which usually takes around 6 to 18 months) as medical removal can leave scarring. If requested, the lesions can however be removed by various medical treatments such as cryotherapy (freezing), diathermy (burning), or curettage (cutting or scraping).

In an HIV-positive person, a large outbreak of molluscum contagiosum may indicate that the immune system is critically weak and it is advisable to seek medical attention.

Scabies is an intensely itchy, contagious skin infestation of the parasitic mite Sarcoptes scabiei. The adult female mite is around 0.4 millimetres (one-sixtieth of an inch) long and barely visible by the human eye, with the male being half that size. Female mites burrow into the outer layer of the skin (stratum croneum) to lay eggs.

Scabies symptoms

Symptoms begin two to six weeks after infection and include:

⇨ burrows that appear as silvery or brown wavy lines up to 15 millimetres (half an inch) in length. The burrows can appear anywhere, but usually occur on the webbing between fingers and toes, on the genitals, around the anus, or on the buttocks, elbows or wrists;

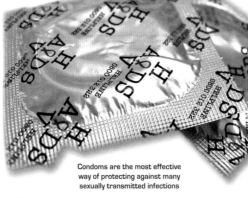

Condoms are the most effective way of protecting against many sexually transmitted infections

⇨ an intensely itchy rash of inflamed pimple-like lumps (papules/lesions) as an allergic reaction to the mites, their eggs and faeces;

⇨ widespread itching, particularly at night or after baths when the body is warmer, as a reaction to the mites.

Again, scabies it not strictly a sex-ually transmitted disease, as the scabies mite can be passed on through other forms of prolonged direct skin contact. Scabies has been known to spread rapidly in crowded conditions where there is frequent contact between people, such as in care homes or childcare facilities. It is also possible, but much less likely, to acquire the infestation through sharing clothes, towels or bedding with someone infected. Sexual activity does, however, carry a particularly high risk of transmission.

There is no effective way to prevent infection apart from avoiding direct skin contact with an infected person. If a person knows that they are infected then they can prevent the infestation spreading by washing clothes and bedding on a hot wash to kill the mites (at 50 degrees Celsius / 120 Fahrenheit or above). Treatment comes in the form of lotions that can be bought from pharmacies without prescription and applied to the body to kill the parasites. It is recommended that all people in close contact, such as sexual partners or members of the household, should be treated at the same time, even if they are not yet showing any symptoms of infestation.

Syphilis is a bacterial infection caused by treponema pallidum, which used to be known as the pox. It is usually sexually transmitted, but can also be passed from an infected woman to her unborn child. Syphilis progresses through several stages, of which the primary and secondary stages are very infectious.

Syphilis symptoms
Syphilis symptoms can be difficult to recognise and may take three months to appear after sexual contact with an infected person. They include:

⇨ one or more painless ulcers on the penis, vagina, vulva, cervix, anus or mouth;

⇨ small lumps in the groin due to swollen glands;

⇨ a non-itchy rash;

⇨ fever or flu-like symptoms.

Left untreated, the infection progresses to a latent stage. This may be followed by tertiary syphilis, which can seriously affect organs such as the heart, sometimes leading to death.

Thrush, also known as candidiasis, is a yeast infection caused by the candida species of fungus. Thrush is not technically a sexually transmitted infection, as candida is a common yeast that is found on the skin and genitals of most people, even those who have not had sex. Candida is usually suppressed by the immune system and the natural bacteria found in the body, but there are many things that can upset the balance and allow candida to grow.

There are at least 25 different sexually transmitted diseases with a range of different symptoms

---

Thrush symptoms
The symptoms of a thrush infection are:

⇨ in women – irritation, itching, thick white discharge, redness, soreness and swelling of the vagina and vulva;

⇨ in men – irritation, discharge from the penis, difficulty pulling back the foreskin usually caused by the swelling of the head of the penis (balanitis). Thrush occurs a lot less frequently in men.

Thrush causes
There are many causes of thrush, but the most common are:

⇨ in women, wearing nylon or lycra clothes that are too tight (the lack of air circulation can cause Candida to proliferate);

⇨ certain antibiotics or contraceptive pills that alter the pH balance of the vagina;

⇨ a change in the hormonal balance in pregnant women, causing a change in the level of normal bacteria;

⇨ spermicides (found on some condoms) or perfumed toiletries that irritate the vagina or penis;

⇨ douching (washing out the vagina) or using tampons;

⇨ sexual contact (either genital or oral) with someone who carries the candida yeast.

Treatment for thrush involves applying an anti-fungal cream that contains Clotrimazole. If an infection is recurring then Fluconazole may be prescribed to be taken orally, unless the patient is pregnant. It may also be suggested to wash the genitals with water only to avoid irritation, use sanitary towels instead of tampons, and wear loose fitting cotton underwear and clothes.

Trichomoniasis (also known as Trich) is caused by the single-celled organism trichomonas vaginalis, which is transmitted through sex. It can infect the vagina and the male and female urethra. Often this STD presents no symptoms, though women are more likely to have symptoms than men.

Trichomoniasis symptoms
If symptoms do appear, they commonly include:

⇨ discharge in both men and women (sometimes copious and unpleasant smelling in women);

⇨ discomfort or pain whilst having sex;

⇨ pain when urinating and inflammation of the urethra.

Women may also experience an inflammation of the vulva and cystitis (an infection of the urinary system).

Transmission is usually through vaginal, anal or oral sex with an infected person. The most effective prevention method is to practise safer sex by using condoms.

Treatment for both men and women is a drug called metronidazole which can be taken orally or applied as a gel. It is important for any sexual partners to also be treated as trichomoniasis can be carried and spread without symptoms. If a woman is pregnant then she should seek medical advice before pursuing treatment.

⇨ The above information is reprinted with kind permission from AVERT. Visit www.avert.org for more information.

© AVERT

Sexually transmitted infections – statistics

Information from the fpa

Statistical sources

United Kingdom (UK) statistics on sexually transmitted infections (STIs) are based on diagnoses made at genitourinary medicine (GUM) clinics.[1] These will underestimate true prevalence as diagnoses made in other healthcare settings such as family planning clinics and general practice are not included, and many infections such as genital Chlamydia and gonorrhea often show no symptoms and remain undiagnosed.

Data for HIV diagnoses and AIDS are collated from a number of surveillance reports across the UK.[2]

General trends

⇨ In a survey of sexual attitudes and lifestyles in Great Britain,[3] 10.8 per cent of men and 12.6 per cent of women aged 16-44 reported ever having a sexually transmitted infection.

⇨ In 2007, there were 397,990 new sexually transmitted infection diagnoses at GUM clinics in the UK, an increase of 63 per cent on 1998.[1]

⇨ Between 2006 and 2007 the number of new diagnoses increased by six per cent.

⇨ Between 1998 and 2007 the largest increases were seen in diagnoses of genital Chlamydia which rose by 150 per cent, genital herpes by 51 per cent and syphilis by 1,828 per cent.

⇨ New cases of gonorrhea in 2007 decreased for the fifth year running.

The overall rise in diagnoses can be attributed to a number of factors including increased transmission, a greater awareness of sexually transmitted infections leading to more people coming forward for testing, improved acceptability of GUM clinics and the development of more sensitive diagnostic tests.

⇨ In 2007, over one million sexual health screens were carried out at GUM clinics in the UK, 10 per cent more than in 2006.

Chlamydia

⇨ Genital Chlamydia remains the most common bacterial sexually transmitted infection seen at GUM clinics in the UK, with 121,986 diagnoses in 2007, a rise of seven per cent since 2006.

⇨ The overall rate of new diagnoses was 201.3 per 100,000 population.

⇨ The highest rates of diagnoses were among women aged 16-19 (1,423 per 100,000) and 20-24 (1,179.3 per 100,000) and men aged 20–24 (1,182.5 per 100,000).

⇨ Young people aged 16-24 years accounted for 65 per cent of all new diagnoses.

⇨ These data do not include cases diagnosed through the national screening programme in England (see below), unless they are referred to GUM clinics for management.

Obtaining accurate estimates of the true prevalence of Chlamydia is difficult as the infection is often asymptomatic and is liable to remain undetected. The Department of Health (DH) began the phased implementation of a National Chlamydia Screening Programme (NCSP) for sexually active women and men under 25 years of age in England in April 2003. By June 2007, over 60 per cent of Primary Care Trusts were actively taking part. Scotland, Wales and Northern Ireland have not set up national Chlamydia screening programmes.

⇨ Between 2003 and 2007, around one in ten of those screened were found to be positive.[4]

⇨ Chlamydia is implicated in more than 50 per cent of cases of pelvic inflammatory disease,[5] which can lead to ectopic pregnancy and infertility in women. It may be associated with fertility problems in men.[6]

Genital warts

⇨ Genital warts are the most common viral sexually transmitted infection diagnosed at GUM clinics in the UK, with 89,838 diagnoses in 2007, a rise of seven per cent since 2006.

⇨ The overall rate of new diagnoses was 148.3 per 100,000 population.

Categories of sexually transmitted infection

Sexually transmitted infections fall into these four categories:

Bacterial	Viral	Parasitic	Fungal
Gonorrhea	HIV (the virus that can lead to AIDS)	Scabies mites	Candida (Thrush)
Chlamydia	Hepatitis A, B, C	Pubic lice	
Syphilis	Genital warts	Trichomoniasis	
Non-specific urethritis	Genital herpes		

How are they cured or treated?

Antibiotics	Antivirals	Lotions	Lotions and antibiotics
Curable	Treatable	Curable	Curable

Source: Cambridge University Students' Union (CUSU)

⇨ The highest rates of diagnoses were in women aged 16-19 (830.1 per 100,000) and men aged 20-24 (815.2 per 100,000).

Diagnoses of genital warts at GUM clinics across the UK have been slowly increasing, and many more cases are likely to be diagnosed and treated in other healthcare settings such as general practice.

Genital warts are the clinical visible manifestation of the human papilloma virus (HPV), mainly types 6 and 11. Some high-risk types of HPV are associated with cervical cancer; however, these rarely show up as visible warts and are likely to remain undiagnosed.

Gonorrhoea

⇨ There were 18,710 diagnoses of gonorrhea at GUM clinics in the UK in 2007, a fall of one per cent since 2006.
⇨ The overall rate of new diagnoses was 30.9 per 100,000.
⇨ The highest rates of diagnoses were in women aged 16-19 (136.9 per 100,000) and men aged 20-24 (174.2 per 100,000).
⇨ Men accounted for 69 per cent of the overall diagnoses, with nearly a third of these occurring in men who have sex with men (MSM).

Rates for gonorrhea are highest in predominantly urban regions, and higher in London (90.3 per 100,000) than any other part of the UK. This is likely to reflect the sub groups most at risk; in the UK these include MSM and black ethnic groups.

Syphilis

⇨ There were 2,680 diagnoses of syphilis at GUM clinics in the UK in 2007, with little change since 2006.
⇨ Men accounted for 89 per cent of the diagnoses; the highest rate occurred in the 25-34 age group (18.3 per 100,000).
⇨ In 2007, 62 per cent of all syphilis diagnoses in males were among MSM.

Although syphilis is still a relatively rare condition, since 1999 there has been a substantial increase in the number of diagnoses mainly due to localised outbreaks, particularly in Bristol, London, Brighton and Manchester. Many of the cases have been among MSM; however, heterosexual men and women have also been affected. Investigations into the outbreaks have shown some common behavioural features, including high rates of partner change and anonymous contacts, unprotected oral sex, recreational drug use during sexual intercourse, and concomitant HIV infection.[7]

Genital herpes

⇨ There were 26,062 diagnoses of genital herpes simplex at GUM clinics in the UK in 2007, an increase of 20 per cent since 2006.
⇨ The overall rate of new diagnoses was 43.0 per 100,000.
⇨ The highest rates of diagnoses were in women aged 16-19 (209.8 per 100,000) and 20-24 (41.9 per 100,000).

Chlamydia remains the most common bacterial sexually transmitted infection seen at GUM clinics in the UK

Diagnoses of genital herpes made at GUM clinics are likely to underestimate true prevalence as many people will be diagnosed and treated in other healthcare settings or may not seek treatment at all.

Genital herpes is caused by the herpes simplex virus (HSV) which has two subtypes, 1 (HSV-1) and 2 (HSV-2). Both types can cause symptoms on the genitals but also on the face (cold sores).[8] Changes in sexual behaviour where oral sex is becoming more common[9] and a decreased immunity in young people to HSV-1[9] have been identified as a contributing factor to a rise in incidence of genital herpes.

HIV/AIDS

By 31 December 2007:[10]
⇨ 6,393 new diagnoses of HIV in the UK had been reported, compared with 7,276 in 2006. Due to delays in reported diagnoses, this figure is expected to rise;

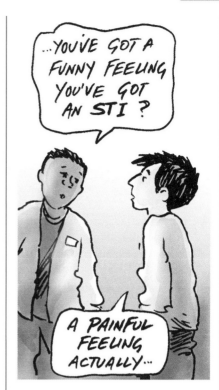

⇨ 43 per cent of infections were acquired through heterosexual intercourse. The majority of these were acquired outside the UK;
⇨ 34 per cent of infections were acquired through sex between men. MSM remain most at risk of acquiring HIV within the UK;
⇨ there were 503 AIDS diagnoses and 445 HIV-related deaths, compared with 1,083 diagnoses and 749 HIV-related deaths in 1997.

By the end of 2007 there were an estimated 73,000 people living with HIV in the UK, of whom about a third had not had their infections diagnosed. Highly active antiretroviral therapies (HAART) have resulted in substantial reductions in AIDS incidence and deaths in the UK, which, in turn, has led to an increase in the number of people needing long-term treatment.

Government policy

Governments in England,[11] Wales[12] and Scotland[13] have all published policy documents which address sexual health issues, including the need to reduce the incidence of sexually transmitted infections. Northern Ireland has a HIV/AIDS policy[14] in place and a sexual health promotion strategy, which was subject to an extensive consultation, is expected to be published soon.[15]

References

1 Health Protection Agency, *STIs annual data*, accessed 6 August 2008.
2 Health Protection Agency, *HIV*, accessed 6 August 2008.
3 Fenton, K. et al, 'Sexual behaviour in Britain: reported sexually transmitted infections and prevalent genital Chlamydia trachomatis infection', *Lancet*, vol 358, (2001), 1851-1854.
4 National Chlamydia Screening Programme, *Maintaining Momentum: Annual report of the National Chlamydia Screening Programme in England, 2006/07* (London: Health Protection Agency, 2007).
5 Moss, T.R. ed, *International Handbook of Chlamydia 2nd ed* (Haslemere: Euromed Communications, 2006).
6 Idahl, A. et al, 'Demonstration of Chlamydia trachomatis IgG antibodies in the male partner of the infertile couple is correlated with a reduced likelihood of achieving pregnancy', *Human Reproduction*, vol 19, (2004), 1121-1126.
7 Doherty, L. et al, 'Syphilis: old problem, new strategy', *BMJ*, vol 325, (2002), 153-156.
8 Adler, M. et al, ABC of *Sexually Transmitted Infections 5th ed* (London: BMJ Books, 2005).
9 Johnson, A.M., 'Sexual behaviour in Britain: partnerships, practices, and HIV risk behaviours', *Lancet*, vol 358, (2001), 1835-1842.
10 Health Protection Agency Centre for Infections et al, *New HIV Diagnoses Surveillance Tables: UK Data to the end of December 2007* (London: HPA, 2007).
11 Department of Health, *National Strategy for Sexual Health and HIV* (London: DH, 2001).
12 National Assembly for Wales, *A Strategic Framework for Promoting Sexual Health in Wales* (Cardiff: National Assembly for Wales, 2000).
13 Scottish Executive, *Respect and Responsibility. Strategy and action plan for improving sexual health* (Edinburgh: Scottish Executive, 2005).
14 Northern Ireland Department of Health and Social Services, *HIV and AIDS in Northern Ireland: A strategy* (Belfast: HMSO, 1993).
15 Northern Ireland Department of Health Social Services and Public Safety, *A Five Year Sexual Health Promotion Strategy and Action Plan. Consultative Document* (Belfast: DHSSPSNI, 2003).
August 2008

⇨ The above information is reprinted with kind permission from **fpa**. Visit www.fpa.org.uk for more information.

© *fpa*

Brits turn a blind eye to STIs

Information from Mintel

With Sexual Health Week now in full flow, new research from Mintel can reveal that attitudes to sexual health are still alarmingly relaxed in Britain today. Indeed, just one in three adults (33%) say they always use a condom with a new partner, a time when it really is important to take precautions. Surprisingly, one in ten Brits (11%) are still too embarrassed to buy condoms – a figure that is just as high amongst older adults as it is amongst Britain's teenagers.

The research also shows that 31% of adults don't use a condom because they trust that their partner does not have a sexually transmitted infection (STI), while the same proportion (32%) simply don't think they are at risk of catching an STI at all.

'It is clear that many Brits have become very blasé about safe sex. Messages about sexual health and protecting against both pregnancy and STIs are not getting through. Communications are either not being clearly delivered, or more dangerously, not being listened to,' comments Katy Child, senior market analyst at Mintel.

What is more, 33% stop using a condom when in a long-term relationship. They assume that a committed relationship reduces the risk of an STI but this is only true if both partners have been tested and cleared of STIs.

'There is still a taboo surrounding STIs that needs addressing. People need to be encouraged to take responsibility for protecting themselves and to speak more openly about these issues with their partners. Using condoms and testing for STIs needs to become the norm and not something to be embarrassed about,' says Katy Child.

According to the figures from Mintel, condom sales and distribution (through shops and the NHS) have remained relatively static since 2003, at around 190 million condoms a year.

The Shirley Valentine effect

Many sexual health awareness campaigns target teenagers and young adults. But today it seems that Britain's over-45s could do with a crash course in these matters. Rising divorce rates and vastly changing attitudes mean that there is now a large number of people of this age getting back on the dating scene. Messaging needs to be as relevant to this age group as it is to the younger generation.

'People coming out of long-term relationships and looking for love again may be unaware of the risks of contracting STIs. Condoms that are marketed specifically to divorcees might just strike a chord,' explains Katy Child.
July 2008

⇨ The above information is reprinted with kind permission from Mintel. Visit www.mintel.com for more information.

© *Mintel*

Breaking the cycle of STIs

Information from the United Nations Population Fund (UNFPA)

Some 340 million new cases of curable sexually transmitted infections (STIs) occur every year. The figure does not include HIV or other viral STIs – including hepatitis B, genital herpes and genital warts, which are not curable.

The most common of the curable STIs are gonorrhea, syphilis, Chlamydia and trichomoniasis. Their prevention and treatment is an important part of UNFPA's mandate, as agreed to at the ICPD. Sexually transmitted infections constitute a significant health burden and increase the risks of transmission of HIV.

Sexually transmitted infections continue to take an enormous toll on health, particularly on women's reproductive health. In fact, next to complications of pregnancy and childbirth, they are the leading cause of health problems for women of reproductive age. They can cause pregnancy-related complications, including spontaneous abortions, premature birth, stillbirth and congenital infections. They can also lead to pelvic inflammatory disease and cervical cancer. Every year, at least half a million infants are born with congenital syphilis. In addition, maternal syphilis causes another half a million stillbirths and miscarriages annually. Most cases of infertility are attributable to STIs.

Women and young people at risk

Worldwide, the disease burden of STIs in women is more than five times that of men. The presence of one or more STIs increases the risk of becoming infected with HIV by two to nine times. Women's greater susceptibility to these infections is based on both biological and social realities. Women's health can also be affected by reproductive health tract infections that are not sexually transmitted, including vaginosis and candida.

Sexually active young people are especially vulnerable to STIs. Each day, some 500,000 young people, mostly young women, are infected with an STI (excluding HIV). Those who become sexually active at an early age are more likely to change sexual partners and risk greater exposure. Most know very little about these infections and many are reluctant to seek services. Only 17 per cent of sexually active young people use contraceptives. Many are unaware that condoms offer dual protection from unwanted pregnancy and STIs. Even if they want to use condoms, they may not have ready access to them, or may be unable to negotiate their use.

Strategies to prevent and treat STIs

UNFPA supports the integration and prevention and treatment of STIs within a package of reproductive services. For instance, screening of pregnant women is an important aspect of antenatal care, as STIs can be dangerous for both mothers and newborns. Making 'youth-friendly' reproductive health information and services readily accessible to young people is another cornerstone of UNFPA's approach to the problem. UNFPA is also active in procurement and logistical support for both male and female condoms.

Other key strategies to combat STIs include:

⇨ condom promotion and distribution;

⇨ community-based advocacy on the dangers of STIs and ways to prevent them;

⇨ early diagnosis and treatment (of clients and their partners);

⇨ providing specific services for populations at risk – such as long-distance truck drivers, military personnel and prisoners.

⇨ The above information is reprinted with kind permission from the United Nations Population Fund (UNFPA). Visit www.unfpa.org for more information.

© United Nations Population Fund (UNFPA)

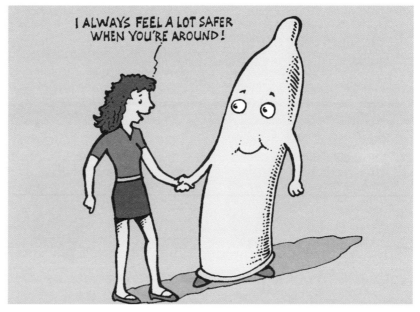

Methods of protection

Information from the Cambridge University Students' Union

The pill is an example of contraception. That's something that prevents pregnancy. However, if you want to protect yourself from Sexually Transmitted Infections, contraception isn't enough – you need a barrier method, something which places a physical barrier to protect you. Some things, like the condom, are contraceptives and barrier methods, but it's important to remember the difference.

Condom

What: Latex penis shaped 'glove' that fits over an erect penis.

How to use: Firstly, check that the condom has the British Standard (kite) Mark and the European Standard (CE) Mark. Also check that its expiry date hasn't passed. The condom needs to be put on just before penetration, to catch any precum. Carefully tear the foil, being careful not to damage the condom – you may find it useful to push the condom to one side of the foil to keep it well clear. Make sure you've got it the right way round (so it can be rolled down the penis) and place it onto the end of an erection, making sure you squeeze the teat – otherwise there'll be nowhere for the semen to go, and the condom may well split. Carefully roll the condom down the shaft of the penis – this can be fun to do together. After ejaculation, hold the condom on to the base of the penis as you withdraw. Carefully remove the condom, wrap in tissue and place in a bin – don't flush down a toilet.

Condoms can't be reused – only use once, and that includes if you come before penetrating.

What it protects against: condoms offer protection against unplanned pregnancy, and when used correctly provide 99% protection from STIs which can be caught during intercourse. They're a simple, quick and easy way to make your sex safer.

Avanti condoms

If you're allergic to latex there are Avanti condoms available, which are non-latex. Some people prefer them as they transfer heat well and don't taste of latex. However, they are much more expensive than latex-based condoms.

Lubes/oil

As condoms (and oral shields and latex gloves) are made of latex, it's important not to use any oil-based substance as oil degrades latex and will stop them being effective. Examples of oil-based substances includes Vaseline, lipstick, lip balm and margarine – if you're wearing lip balm and give oral sex to a man wearing a condom, or have greasy hands from your pizza and use them to put the condom on, it might not work properly if you have intercourse after, so BE CAREFUL. To be safe, only used water-based lube such as KY Jelly.

Extra thick and naturelle

Condoms are available in different strengths, naturelle and extra strong.

It used to be the recommendation that extra thick be used for anal sex, although now the official line is that any kitemarked condom is ok. Some may choose to use extra strong condoms for all types of intercourse, as their thickness can help men last longer before orgasm.

Femidom

What: a 'reverse condom' which fits inside the vagina or anus.

How to use: insert before penetration by squeezing the ring in the closed end so it becomes long and thin. Slowly insert and release so that the ring expands. Make sure that the penis is inserted into the femidom, and not to the side.

What it protects against: STIs that can be prevented by using a barrier method.

Oral shield

What: a thin square of latex (although non-latex versions are available).

How to use: place over the area you're making contact with (the vagina for oral sex, the anus for rimming) and use it as a barrier between your tongue and your partner.

What it protects against: STIs that can be prevented by using a barrier method.

Latex glove

What: a thin glove made of latex.

How to use: wear for activities such as fisting or fingering.

What it protects against: STIs that can be prevented by using a barrier method.

There are many methods of contraception, such as the cap and the pill. However, it's important to remember that these offer no protection against STIs.

⇨ The above information is reprinted with kind permission from the Cambridge University Students' Union. Visit www.cusu.cam.ac.uk for more information.

© Cambridge University Students' Union

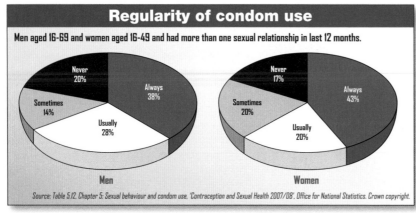

Regularity of condom use

Men aged 16-69 and women aged 16-49 and had more than one sexual relationship in last 12 months.

Men
- Never 20%
- Always 38%
- Sometimes 14%
- Usually 28%

Women
- Never 17%
- Always 43%
- Sometimes 20%
- Usually 20%

Source: Table 5.12, Chapter 5: Sexual behaviour and condom use, 'Contraception and Sexual Health 2007/08', Office for National Statistics. Crown copyright.

Pill still the most popular form of birth control

Women prefer to use the pill ahead of other forms of contraceptive, according to a new survey by the Office for National Statistics

In 2007/08, three-quarters of women in the 16-49 age group reported using some form of contraception, with 28 per cent of women using the pill, compared with 24 per cent who relied on the male condom.

One quarter of women said they did not use any form of contraception in 2007/08, with the most common reason being that they were not in a heterosexual relationship (14 per cent). Three per cent said they were not using contraceptives because they wanted to become pregnant.

The annual survey is carried out on behalf of the NHS Information Centre for health and social care. Questions were addressed to women aged 16-49 and men aged 16-69, and most respondents used a self-completion format.

Other key findings for 2007/08 include:

Emergency contraception

Almost all women (91 per cent) questioned in the survey had heard of hormonal emergency contraception – the 'morning after pill' – but fewer (37 per cent) were aware of the emergency intrauterine device.

Fewer than half of women were correctly aware that the 'morning after pill' remains effective up to 72 hours after intercourse. Eight per cent knew correctly that the emergency IUD was effective up to five days after intercourse.

Six per cent of women believed, incorrectly, that the morning after pill protected them against pregnancy until the next period.

Sexual behaviour

Most men (92 per cent) said they only had sex with women, while one per cent said they only had sex with men. Just under two per cent said they had sex with men and women.

Within all age groups between 20 and 49, a higher percentage of men than women reported multiple sexual partners while, in most age groups, proportionately more women than men reported having had just one partner.

Knowledge of sexually transmitted diseases

Around a half of men (57 per cent) and of women (50 per cent) reported making no changes to their behaviour as a result of what they had heard about HIV/AIDS and other STIs. However, 34 per cent of men and 37 per cent of women said they had increased their use of condoms.

Television programmes were the most commonly mentioned source of information about STIs (31 per cent) followed by television advertisements (22 per cent) and newspapers, magazines or books (20 per cent). The Internet was rarely used as a source of information about STIs, even by young people.

The percentage of people who recognised that Chlamydia is an STI has increased sharply since the question was first asked in 2000/01 – from 35 per cent to 85 per cent for men, and from 65 per cent to 93 per cent for women.

28 October 2008

⇨ The above information is reprinted with kind permission from the Office for National Statistics. Visit www.statistics.gov.uk for more information.

© *Crown copyright 2008.*

Current use of contraception by women

Current use of contraception among women aged 16 to 49, 2007/08.

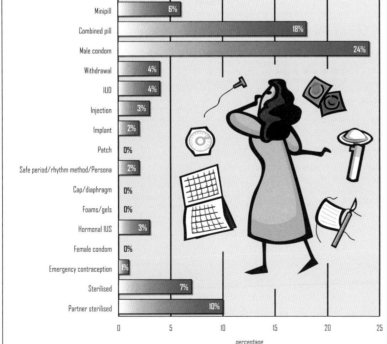

	percentage
Minipill	6%
Combined pill	18%
Male condom	24%
Withdrawal	4%
IUD	4%
Injection	3%
Implant	2%
Patch	0%
Safe period/rhythm method/Persona	2%
Cap/diaphragm	0%
Foams/gels	0%
Hormonal IUS	3%
Female condom	0%
Emergency contraception	1%
Sterilised	7%
Partner sterilised	10%

Source: Table 2.1, Chapter 2: Contraceptive use among women aged under 50, 'Contraception and Sexual Health 2007/08'. Office for National Statistics. Crown copyright.

Pitfalls of condom use

Information from Cambridge University Students' Union

There are several reasons that condoms fail – and in the vast majority of cases it's down to them being used wrongly. Here are some tips on how to minimise the risk of that happening.

⇨ Safety marks: Only ever use condoms with the British Kite Mark and the European Safety Standard – this means that the condom was tested for 'vigorous vaginal intercourse', and passed. If you've got a slightly wacky condom (glow in the dark, or from a novelty shop) this is how to tell if it is safe to use, or only a toy.

⇨ Storage: Make sure you store your condoms well. Don't put them anywhere where they'll be exposed to a wide range of temperatures – especially not in direct sunlight. Don't keep them in your wallet or pocket, as the heat and pressure will cause them to degrade quicker and so the expiry date will be wrong.

⇨ Expiry date: Always check the expiry date. They're often years into the future, but if you find some you'd forgotten you had, check they haven't been sitting there for too long!

⇨ Lube: Make sure that nothing oil-based could come into contact with latex based condoms – and that includes lip balm and chip grease. In the heat of the moment, it's possible you'll reach for all sorts of strange things – make sure they're not oil-based like butter, massage oil, Vaseline...

⇨ Practice: Practise makes perfect, and if you've never used a condom before then it's a good idea to try by yourself first. It also means that you'll know what it feels like, and it's less likely that you'll ejaculate prematurely.

Many people misuse condoms when they've had too much to drink, or are on drugs. Here are some tips on staying in control when you're out for a night:

⇨ eat something before you start drinking;

⇨ only take out as much money as you'll need – including a taxi;

⇨ start off with a big soft drink;

⇨ alternate between non-alcoholic and alcoholic drinks;

⇨ take as much time as you'd like – don't try to keep up;

⇨ avoid getting into rounds;

⇨ avoid crisps and peanuts – they make you thirsty;

⇨ go home when you've reached your limit;

⇨ watch your drink and don't leave it unattended; drink spiking does happen, don't let it happen to you.

⇨ The above information is re-printed with kind permission from Cambridge University Students' Union. Visit www.cusu.cam.ac.uk for more information.

© Cambridge University Students' Union

STI testing

Information from Teens First for Health

If you have had unprotected sex (oral, vaginal or anal sex without using a condom) there is a chance that you may have caught a sexually transmitted infection (STI) such as Chlamydia, gonorrhea, herpes or even HIV.

If you have symptoms that make you think you may have an STI it is really important to go and get it treated. Otherwise you may risk passing it on to other people. Common symptoms include an abnormal discharge from the penis or vagina, pain on passing urine, and developing new lumps or a painful sore in the genital area. However, some infections have no symptoms at all so the only way to find out if you carry the infection is to have a sexual health check-up.

Where do I go?

You can either have tests for STIs done at your local general practice (though you may have to ask in advance) or at the GUM (genito-urinary medicine) clinic at your local hospital. Many young people prefer to visit GUM clinics as they often offer clinic services specifically for young people. If you are under 16 you can attend the clinic on your own. The doctor or nurse who sees you will keep all your medical details confidential and will not tell your GP or parents anything without your permission. The health professionals seeing you are obliged to make your safety and wellbeing their main concern.

Visit the RU Thinking website (www.ruthinking.co.uk) to find a GUM clinic. The clinic may ask a few general questions when you phone up to make an appointment so if you have symptoms or know that

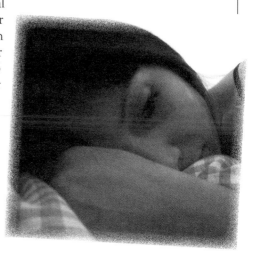

your regular partner has an STI you must make sure to tell them. A lot of young person's clinics are walk-in services, which means you don't need to make an appointment but have to be prepared to wait to be seen.

What will happen?
You will be asked to fill in a registration form when you arrive (you don't even have to leave your real name if you don't want to). When you have done this you will been seen by a doctor or nurse. They will ask you your reasons for wanting a test and some personal questions about your sex life. These questions can be a bit embarrassing but you really should tell them the truth. These doctors speak to people about their sex lives every working day so it would be pretty difficult to shock them!

Some infections have no symptoms at all so the only way to find out if you carry the infection is to have a sexual health check-up

---

After talking to the doctor or nurse you may need to be examined.
For girls:
Tests for infection will be taken from your vagina, cervix (the neck of your womb), urethra (urinary opening) and if necessary your bottom and your throat (depending if you have had anal or oral sex). These are usually cotton tip swabs and small plastic loops, the trick is to try and relax during the examination. The person examining you will explain exactly what they are going to do. If you feel nervous you can ask for a nurse chaperone or a friend to come in the room with you to keep you company.
For boys:
Swabs will be taken from your urethra (urinary opening at end of penis) and if necessary your bottom and your throat (depending if you have had oral sex or received anal sex). You may also be asked to give a urine sample to test for Chlamydia (this needs to be fresh so there is no point bringing a sample with you). The clinic will

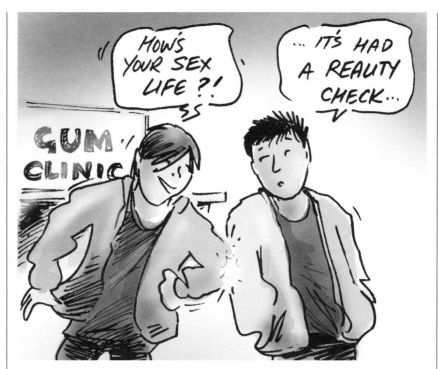

want you to not pass urine for at least two hours before your tests are done, so don't go to the loo when you get to the clinic until you have been seen. The urethra test is only a bit uncomfortable, so don't worry that the tests will be painful and let that put you off having a check-up!

What will they test for?
The standard test clinics include tests for:
⇨ Chlamydia (swab or urine test);
⇨ gonorrhea (swab);
⇨ warts;
⇨ herpes;
⇨ HIV/AIDs;
⇨ hepatitis.
   You will also be offered blood tests to diagnose:
⇨ HIV/AIDS;
⇨ hepatitis;
⇨ syphilis.

Who will examine me?
A doctor or nurse will examine you. If you feel uncomfortable being examined by someone of a different gender to yourself, it is your right to ask for a clinician of the same sex. Girls being examined by a male doctor will always have a female chaperone present. If you would like to be examined by someone of the same sex it is often a good idea to phone up in advance to check that there will be a female/male clinician working that day.

How long will it take?
This will depend on the tests that you need and whether you have an appointment or visit a drop-in clinic. If necessary, call the clinic beforehand and ask for an estimated time.

When will I find out the results?
Some tests will be given to you after a short wait. For some tests, microscopes on site can be used to look at the swabs. These will be done while you wait. Other tests need to be sent off to a lab. You will have to phone later in the week to hear about these. If necessary you may have to go back for treatment.

Treatments
The GUM clinic will provide you with free treatments for STIs if you need them. These are usually tablets, pessaries and creams.
   At GUM clinics, you can also get free condoms and sexual health advice.
   Gay and bisexual men may also be able to have a free hepatitis B vaccination.

⇨ This article has been reproduced with kind permission from Children First for Health – Great Ormond Street Hospital's leading health information website for young people of all ages and parents: www.childrenfirst.nhs.uk
© Great Ormond Street Hospital

'Nice girls' refuse to get checked for STIs

Information from Lloyds Pharmacy

⇨ **66 per cent of those at risk of STIs refuse to go to a clinic.**

⇨ **Women think 'nice girls' don't get STIs.**

⇨ **Lloydspharmacy launches regulated online Chlamydia test service.**

Two-thirds of people who are at risk of contracting sexually transmitted infections* have never attended a GUM clinic and said they wouldn't do so unless they were suffering from symptoms.

The findings are revealed today by Lloydspharmacy to launch its new service: Online Doctor at http://onlinedoctor.lloydspharmacy.com

The new online service offers screening and treatment for chlamydia. One in ten sexually active people are thought to have the infection in the UK.

Of those who said they had not attended a clinic, over half said it was because they were too embarrassed. Women in particular said they were paranoid about being seen by family and friends entering or leaving the clinic. Many women said they thought clinics might be unsavoury places and that, in any case, 'nice girls don't get STIs'.

How the online Chlamydia test works

After registering with the service, men and women receive a vial for a urine sample through the post. They then simply post the sample to a laboratory in a pre-paid envelope. The result will be available in around 48 hours. This will be reviewed by a GP. If the test is positive, a prescription for an antibiotic can be sent directly to the patient's home or preferred address.

According to the research, 76 per cent of sexually active people under 50 who are not in a long-term relationship said that they do not discuss their sexual history with new or current partners and 89 per cent said they would not tell new or current partners if they had contracted an STI in the past.

Chris Frost, Head of Medicines at Lloydspharmacy, says that the stigma and embarrassment surrounding STIs means that new ways of reaching people are needed.

'Unfortunately nice people do indeed get STIs, and the figures for Chlamydia show that most who are infected don't know it until it's too late.'

> **According to the research, 76 per cent of sexually active people under 50 who are not in a long-term relationship said that they do not discuss their sexual history with new or current partners**

The Lloydspharmacy service is perfect for people who would ordinarily be too shy to buy testing kits in store or visit a clinic. The online service was launched on the 16 July and only offers Chlamydia testing currently, but the range of services and prescriptions will grow over time.

The Lloydspharmacy service is supplied by the only Healthcare Commission-regulated online registered GP service, Dr Thom, who will review the lab results of all tests before a prescription can be dispensed.
August 2008

⇨ The above information is reprinted with kind permission from Lloydspharmacy. Visit www.lloydspharmacy.com for more.

© Lloyds Pharmacy

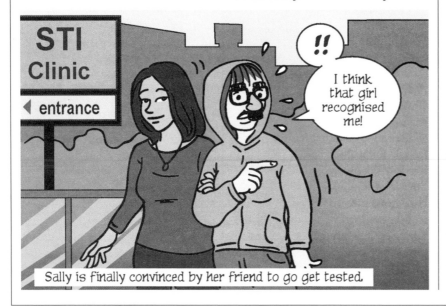

Sally is finally convinced by her friend to go get tested.

Benefits of school-based clinics

The benefits for young people of sexual health services on the school or college site

Private and confidential

Young people give confidentiality top priority when deciding whether or not to use a service. The benefit of on-site sexual health services is that young people can use the service in a place which is young-people centred and offers privacy.

Being able to access confidential sexual health services during the day, at lunch time or during free periods makes it easy for young people to use services discreetly.

Flexibility and access

Policy reforms in health make a strong argument for more flexible services for young people. Locating sexual health services in the places where young people learn provides this flexibility.

Young people in rural areas travel long distances to school or college – at least 50 miles in some cases – so services provided on-site may be their only option.

Developing skills

For many young people their only experience of using health services will have been accompanied by a parent or guardian. Using a service independently for the first time can be daunting. Education institutions are well-placed to build young people's confidence in accessing health services both on and off-site.

In schools: PSHE teachers, learning mentors, Connexions PAs and the school nurse can help by telling young people about what services are available and how to access them.

In further education settings: tutors, youth workers and student support officers can help overcome the barriers of fear and stigma that may prevent young people from accessing services.

The non-medical environment of school- or college-based sexual health services is more comfortable. It encourages young people to go and talk about problems and ask questions early on rather than to only use services when they consider themselves to be 'ill'.

A positive experience of accessing a service can set a pattern for life.

Young men

Evidence shows that young men are more likely to access sexual health services based in school or college than to go to a community clinic or their GP.

Nationally, young men made up only 18% of young people testing in the Chlamydia screening programme in 2005. But where testing has been offered in further education settings at least 50% of those testing were young men.

Schools report equal use of on-site sexual health services by young men and young women. In some cases, young men outnumber young women.

⇨ The above information is taken from the Sex Education Forum website page 'The benefits for young people of sexual health services on the school or college site', and is reprinted with kind permission from NCB. Visit www.ncb.org.uk/sef for more information.

© *National Children's Bureau*

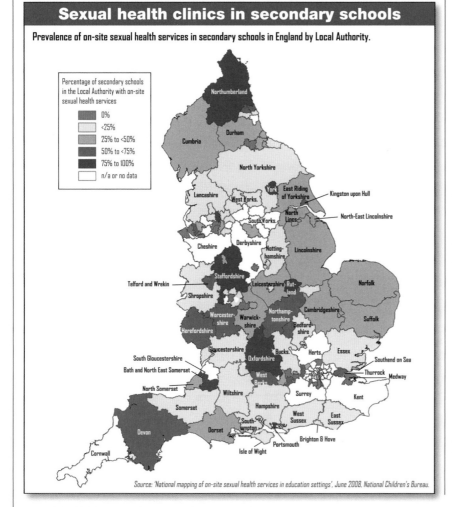

Sexual health clinics in secondary schools

Prevalence of on-site sexual health services in secondary schools in England by Local Authority.

Percentage of secondary schools in the Local Authority with on-site sexual health services
- 0%
- <25%
- 25% to <50%
- 50% to <75%
- 75% to 100%
- n/a or no data

Source: 'National mapping of on-site sexual health services in education settings', June 2008. National Children's Bureau.

School clinics could reduce pregnancy and infection

Information from the University of the West of England

Young people are more likely to use sexual health services if they can access them at schools, according to research by the University of the West of England. A pilot scheme offering drop-in sexual health clinics in Bristol schools has successfully accessed 'hard to reach' groups including boys and vulnerable young people who would not otherwise have received advice.

The outreach scheme was run by Brook in partnership with Bristol City Council and Bristol Primary Care Trust in 16 schools in Neighbourhood Renewal areas of Bristol. It was set up in response to a 143% rise nationally in sexually trans-mitted diseases between 1991 and 2001, and the Department of Health's UK Sexual Health Strategy aimed at reducing the rates of pregnancy and sexually transmitted diseases in the under 18 age group.

Young people using the service reacted very positively to it, and said that the approachability and accessibility of staff was key to its success. The report's author Debra Salmon, of UWE's Faculty of Health and Life Sciences, said, '61% of the young people we surveyed said they attended because it was at school and easy to access and that they would not have attended alternative provision.'

Melanie Iddon of Brook said, 'Brook's approach is to take services to young people, because we believe that's the most effective way of engaging and supporting them. We know that outreach work like this also provides an effective bridge to clinic-based services. We're delighted that the research has endorsed this approach and shown how effective it can be simply to provide services where they're most needed.'

Nurses or youth workers provided advice and treatment including contraception, emergency contraception, pregnancy testing and advice, testing and treatment for sexually transmitted infections and other health-related issues. The multi-disciplinary nature of the team was another reason for the success – youth workers were key in preventive work and talking to young men.

Councillor Peter Hammond, Deputy Leader of Bristol City Council and Executive Member for Cohesion and Raising Attainment, said: 'The findings of this research show how important it is for young people to have access to advice and help with sexual health issues in a setting that is convenient to them. Parents should be reassured that the confidential service will always include advice that young people should talk to their parents about their situation.

'Reducing teenage pregnancy rates is part of our drive to raise standards in schools. It is vital we keep children in school and focused on their education.'

Key findings of the evaluation include:

⇨ Attendances rose to around 1500 per quarter during the 15-month period of the evaluation.

⇨ The ratio of boys to girls attending was 38% to 62%.

⇨ The ratio of boys rose to 48% when youth workers as well as nurses were available to give advice.

⇨ The school-based service provided signposting to other services available.

⇨ Clinic staff supported schools by providing specialist input for school Personal, Social and Health Education sessions.

⇨ The health outcomes for those attending for contraception were good in relation to prevention of pregnancy and early identification of sexually transmitted infections.

Hugh Annett, Director of Public Health, Bristol Primary Care Trust, said: 'The Brook 4YP Service is an outstanding example of partnership working delivering to young people. This was a pilot project supported by the City Council using Neighbourhood Renewal funding. It was rigorously evaluated, shown to be successful and then continued and expanded using PCT funds. It is and will make a significant contribution to improving the sexual health of young people in Bristol.'
10 June 2008

⇨ The above information is reprinted with kind permission from the University of the West of England. Visit www.uwe.ac.uk for more information.
© University of the West of England

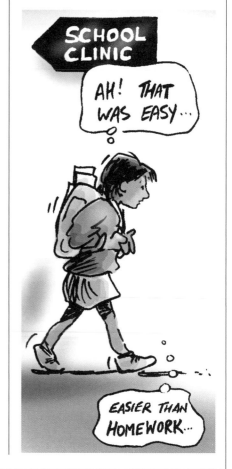

Sex education that works

Information from AVERT

What is sex education?

Sex education, which is sometimes called sexuality education or sex and relationships education, is the process of acquiring information and forming attitudes and beliefs about sex, sexual identity, relationships and intimacy. Sex education is also about developing young people's skills so that they make informed choices about their behaviour, and feel confident and competent about acting on these choices. It is widely accepted that young people have a right to sex education, partly because it is a means by which they are helped to protect themselves against abuse, exploitation, unintended pregnancies, sexually transmitted diseases and HIV/AIDS.

What are the aims of sex education?

Sex education seeks both to reduce the risks of potentially negative outcomes from sexual behaviour, like unwanted or unplanned pregnancies and infection with sexually transmitted diseases, and to enhance the quality of relationships. It is also about developing young people's ability to make decisions over their lifetime. Sex education that works, by which we mean that it is effective, is sex education that contributes to this overall aim.

What skills should sex education develop?

If sex education is going to be effective it needs to include opportunities for young people to develop skills, as it can be hard for them to act on the basis of only having information. The skills young people develop as part of sex education are linked to more general life-skills. Being able to communicate, listen, negotiate, ask for and identify sources of help and advice, are useful life-skills and can be applied in terms of sexual relationships. Effective sex education develops young people's skills in negotiation, decision-making, assertion and listening. Other important skills include being able to recognise pressures from other people and to resist them, dealing with and challenging prejudice and being able to seek help from adults – including parents, carers and professionals – through the family, community and health and welfare services. Sex education that works also helps equip young people with the skills to be able to differentiate between accurate and inaccurate information, and to discuss a range of moral and social issues and perspectives on sex and sexuality, including different cultural attitudes and sensitive issues like sexuality, abortion and contraception.

Forming attitudes and beliefs

Young people can be exposed to a wide range of attitudes and beliefs in relation to sex and sexuality. These sometimes appear contradictory and confusing. For example, some health messages emphasise the risks and dangers associated with sexual activity and some media coverage promotes the idea that being sexually active makes a person more attractive and mature. Because sex and sexuality are sensitive subjects, young people and sex educators can have strong views on what attitudes people should hold, and what moral framework should govern people's behaviour – these too can sometimes seem to be at odds. Young people are very interested in the moral and cultural frameworks that binds sex and sexuality. They often welcome opportunities to talk about issues where people have strong views, like abortion, sex before marriage, lesbian and gay issues and contraception and birth control. It is important to remember that talking in a balanced way about differences in opinion does not promote one set of views over another, or mean that one agrees with a particular view. Part of exploring and understanding cultural, religious and moral views is finding out that you can agree to disagree.

People providing sex education have attitudes and beliefs of their own about sex and sexuality and it is important not to let these influence negatively the sex education that they provide. For example, even if a person believes that young people should not have sex until they are married, this does not imply withholding important information about safer sex and contraception. Attempts to impose narrow moralistic views about sex and sexuality on young people through sex education have failed. Rather than trying to deter or frighten young people away from having sex, effective sex education includes work on attitudes and beliefs, coupled with skills development, that enables young people to choose whether or not to have a sexual relationship taking into account the potential risks of any sexual activity.

Effective sex education also provides young people with an opportunity to explore the reasons why people have sex, and to think about how it involves emotions, respect for oneself and other people and their feelings, decisions and bodies. Young people should have the chance to explore gender differences and how ethnicity and sexuality can influence people's feelings and options. They should be able to decide for themselves what the positive qualities of relationships are. It is important that they understand how bullying, stereotyping, abuse and exploitation can negatively influence relationships.

So what information should be given to young people?

Young people get information about sex and sexuality from a wide range of sources including each other, through the media including advertising, television and magazines, as well as leaflets, books and websites (such as www.avert.org) which are intended to be sources of information about sex and sexuality. Some of this will be accurate and some inaccurate.

Providing information through sex education is therefore about finding out what young people already know, adding to their existing knowledge and correcting any misinformation they may have. For example, young people may have heard that condoms are not effective against HIV/AIDS or that there is a cure for AIDS. It is important to provide information which corrects mistaken beliefs. Without correct information young people can put themselves at greater risk.

Information is also important as the basis on which young people can developed well-informed attitudes and views about sex and sexuality. Young people need to have information on all the following topics:

⇨ Sexual development;
⇨ Reproduction;
⇨ Contraception;
⇨ Relationships.

They need to have information about the physical and emotional changes associated with puberty and sexual reproduction, including fertilisation and conception, and about sexually transmitted diseases, including HIV/AIDS. They also need to know about contraception and birth control, including what contraceptives there are, how they work, how people use them, how they decide what to use or not, and how they can be obtained. In terms of information about relationships they need to know about what kinds of relationships there are, about love and commitment, marriage and partnership and the law relating to sexual behaviour and relationships as well as the range of religious and cultural views on sex and sexuality and sexual diversity. In addition, young people should be provided with information about abortion, sexuality and confidentiality, as well as about the range of sources of advice and support that are available in the community and nationally.

When should sex education start?

Sex education that works starts early, before young people reach puberty, and before they have developed established patterns of behaviour. The precise age at which information should be provided depends on the physical, emotional and intellectual development of the young people as well as their level of understanding. What is covered and also how depends on who is providing the sex education, when they are providing it and in what context, as well as what the individual young person wants to know about.

It is important not to delay providing information to young people but to begin when they are young. Providing basic information provides the foundation on which more complex knowledge is built up over time. This also means that sex education has to be sustained. For example, when they are very young, children can be informed about how people grow and change over time, and how babies become children and then adults, and this provides the basis on which they understand more detailed information about puberty provided in the pre-teenage years. They can also, when they are young, be provided with information about viruses and germs that attack the body. This provides the basis for talking to them later about infections that can be caught through sexual contact.

Some people are concerned that providing information about sex and sexuality arouses curiosity and can lead to sexual experimentation. There is no evidence that this happens. It is important to remember that young people can store up information provided at any time, for a time when they need it later on.

Sometimes it can be difficult for adults to know when to raise issues, but the important thing is to maintain an open relationship with children which provides them with opportunities to ask questions when they have them. Parents and carers can also be proactive and engage young people in discussions about sex, sexuality and relationships. Naturally, many parents and their children feel embarrassed about talking about some aspects of sex and sexuality. Viewing sex education as an on-going conversation about values, attitudes and issues as well as providing facts can be helpful. The best basis to proceed on is a sound relationship in which a young person feels able to ask a question or raise an issue if they feel they need to. It has been shown that in countries like the Netherlands, where many families regard it as an important responsibility to talk openly with children about sex and sexuality, this contributes to greater cultural openness about sex and sexuality and improved sexual health among young people.

The role of many parents and carers as sex educators changes as young people get older and young people are provided with more opportunities to receive formal sex education through schools and community settings. However, it doesn't get any less important. Because sex education in school tends to take place in blocks of time, it can't always address issues relevant to young people at a particular time, and parents can fulfil a particularly important role in providing information and opportunities to discuss things as they arise.

Who should provide sex education?

Different settings provide different contexts and opportunities for sex education. At home, young people can easily have one-to-one discussions with parents or carers which focus on specific issues, questions or concerns. They can have a dialogue about their attitudes and views. Sex education at home also tends to take place over a long time, and involve lots of short interactions between parents and children. There may be times when young people seem reluctant to talk, but it is important not to interpret any diffidence as meaning that there is nothing left to talk about. As young people get older, advantage can be taken of opportunities provided by things seen on television, for example, as an opportunity to initiate conversation. It is also important not to defer dealing with a question or issue for too long as it can suggest that you are unwilling to talk about it.

In school, the interaction between the teacher and young people takes a different form and sex education is often provided in organised blocks of lessons. It is not as well-suited to advising the individual as it is to providing information from an impartial point of view. The most effective sex education acknowledges the different contributions each setting can make. School programmes which involve parents, notifying them what is being taught and when, can support the initiation of dialogue at home. Parents and schools both need to engage with young people about the messages that they get from the media, and give them opportunities for discussion.

In some countries, the involvement of young people themselves in developing and providing sex education has increased as a means of ensuring the relevance and accessibility of provision. Consultation with young people at the point when programmes are designed helps ensure that they are relevant and the involvement of young people in delivering programmes may reinforce messages as they model attitudes and behaviour to their peers.

Effective school-based sex education

School-based sex education can be an important and effective way of enhancing young people's knowledge, attitudes and behaviour. There is widespread agreement that formal education should include sex education and what works has been well-researched. Evidence suggests that effective school programmes will include the following elements:

⇨ a focus on reducing specific risky behaviours;
⇨ A basis in theories which explain what influences people's sexual choices and behaviour;
⇨ a clear and continuously re-inforced message about sexual behaviour and risk reduction;
⇨ providing accurate information about the risks associated with sexual activity, contraception and birth control and methods of avoiding or deferring intercourse;
⇨ dealing with peer and other social pressures on young people; providing opportunities to practise communication, negotiation and assertion skills;
⇨ uses a variety of approaches to teaching and learning that involve and engage young people and help them to personalise the information;
⇨ uses approaches to teaching and learning which are appropriate to young people's age, experience and cultural background;
⇨ is provided by people who believe in what they are saying and have access to support in the form of training or consultation with other sex educators.

Formal programmes with these elements have been shown to increase young people's levels of knowledge about sex and sexuality, put back the average age at which they first have sexual intercourse and decrease risk when they do have sex. All the elements are important and inter-related, and sex education needs to be supported by links to sexual health services, otherwise it is not going to be so effective. It also takes into account the messages about sexual values and behaviour young people get from other sources, like friends and the media. It is also responsive to the needs of the young people themselves – whether they are girls or boys, on their own or in a single-sex or mixed-sex group, and what they know already, their age and experiences.

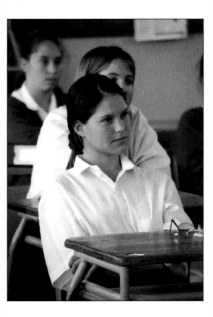

Taking sex education forward

Providing effective sex education can seem daunting because it means tackling potentially sensitive issues. However, because sex education comprises many individual activities which take place across a wide range of settings and periods of time, there are lots of opportunities to contribute.

The nature of a person's contrib-ution depends on their relationship, role and expertise in relation to young people. For example, parents are best placed in relation to young people to provide continuity of individual support and education starting from early in their lives. School-based education programmes are particularly good at providing information and opportunities for skills development and attitude clarification in more formal ways, through lessons within a curriculum. Community-based projects provide opportunities for young people to access advice and information in less formal ways. Sexual health and other health and welfare services can provide access to specific information, support and advice. Sex education through the mass media, often supported by local, regional or national Government and non-governmental agencies and departments, can help to raise public awareness of sexual health issues.

Further development of sex ed-ucation partly depends on joining up these elements in a coherent way to meet the needs of young people. There is also a need to pay more attention to the needs of specific groups of young people like young parents and young lesbian, gay and bisexual people, as well as those who may be out of touch with services and schools and socially vulnerable, like young refugees and asylum-seekers, young people in care, young people in prisons, and also those living on the street.

The circumstances and context available to parents and other sex educators are different from place to place. Practical or political realities in a particular country may limit people's ability to provide young people with comprehensive sex education combining all the elements in the best way possible. But the basic principles outlined here apply everywhere. By making our own contribution and valuing that made by others, and by being guided by these principles, we can provide more sex education that works and improve the support we offer to young people.
Updated 20 February 2009

⇨ The above information is re-printed with kind permission from AVERT. Visit www.avert.org for more information.
© AVERT

Where do baby rabbits come from?

Sex education to begin at five in all schools

⇨ *No opt-out for faith schools, says minister.*
⇨ *Decision welcomed by sexual health campaigners.*

Sex education is to be made a compulsory part of the national curriculum in primary and secondary schools under government plans to cut teenage pregnancies and sexually transmitted infections.

All children in state schools in England will learn about body parts and animal reproduction from the age of five, puberty and intercourse from the age of seven and pregnancy, contraception and safer sex from the age of 11. The new curriculum will attempt to stop sex education being consigned to biology lessons and ensure that children learn about relationships and the option of abstinence along with the facts of life.

Ministers indicated that schools would not be allowed to opt out of the rules. Faith schools will receive separate guidance on how to provide sex and relationship education – which will include contraception, abortion and homosexuality – alongside conflicting religious beliefs.

Jim Knight, the schools minister, said he wanted all schools to teach children more about sex in the context of relationships, including marriage and civil partnerships. He said he hoped better education would help teenagers make more informed decisions about when to have sex and delay losing their virginity. But he denied that the lessons would include learning about specific sexual activities from a very young age.

'We are not talking about five-year-olds being taught about sex. At key stage one [ages five to seven] they will be learning about themselves, their differences, their friendships, how to have strong friendships and how to manage their feelings.'

By Polly Curtis, Education Editor

Secondary schools currently only have to teach the mechanics of sex in biology classes, and not in conjunction with relationships and sexual health. Most schools teach personal, social and health education (PSHE) but it is not compulsory and quality is highly variable.

A recent survey of pupils revealed that four in ten had received no sex education at school.

England has some of the highest rates of teenage pregnancy in Europe and sexually transmitted diseases such as Chlamydia are soaring. Wales and Northern Ireland already have compulsory sex education.

The new compulsory PSHE curriculum, expected by 2010, will also include learning about the risk of drugs and alcohol, how to manage money and how to maintain a healthy diet. Parents should be informed about the contents of sex education classes, Knight said. There will be

a drive to improve the teaching of classes, using dedicated teachers and training.

The government's announcement follows recommendations in an independent review undertaken by representatives from groups spanning the sexual health charities as well as faith groups and schools.

A recent survey of pupils revealed that four in ten had received no sex education at school

A new review led by Sir Alasdair MacDonald, an east London head-teacher, will investigate further how to implement the plan and consider whether parents or even schools should be given an opt-out where there is a religious or moral objection. But Knight said: 'We wouldn't be suggesting a statutory programme of study if we thought schools would have an opt-out.

'There are some that argue having an opt-out for parents for the national curriculum is difficult, but I think it

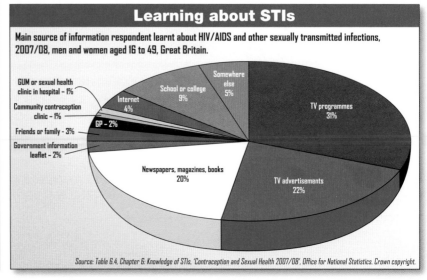

Learning about STIs

Main source of information respondent learnt about HIV/AIDS and other sexually transmitted infections, 2007/08, men and women aged 16 to 49, Great Britain.

- GUM or sexual health clinic in hospital – 1%
- Community contraception clinic – 1%
- GP – 2%
- Friends or family – 3%
- Government information leaflet – 2%
- Internet 4%
- School or college 9%
- Somewhere else 5%
- TV programmes 31%
- TV advertisements 22%
- Newspapers, magazines, books 20%

Source: Table 6.4, Chapter 6: Knowledge of STIs, 'Contraception and Sexual Health 2007/08', Office for National Statistics. Crown copyright.

is important that individual parents' views are taken into account and their right to withdraw because of personal or moral views is respected. It's something it would take a lot for us to move away from.'

He said that supplementary guidance would be produced for Catholic schools advising them that they too must teach all elements of the curriculum alongside Catholic values about contraception, abortion and homosexuality.

The Catholic Education Service denied that this could result in mixed messages for pupils if they were being taught the facts of contraception, then that it was frowned upon. Oona Stannard, director of the CES, said: 'Young people have a right to have age-appropriate information. We can similarly ensure that they are taught the values of their religious faith.'

Sexual health campaigners were thrilled that decades of campaigning for compulsory sex education had come to fruition. Julie Bentley, chief executive of **fpa**, formerly the Family Planning Association, said: 'This is a momentous decision. This move will dramatically improve the long-term health and wellbeing of our children and young people.'

Simon Blake, chief executive of the sexual health charity Brook, said it was an 'absolutely brilliant' move. 'It shows a progressive and bold government that has taken notice of the views of children and young people.'

However, a minority of traditional family campaigners opposed the decision. Stephen Green, national director of Christian Voice, said the proposals would only 'encourage experimentation' and contribute to the rise in teenage pregnancy and infertility.

Headteachers launched an outspoken attack on the plans. John Dunford, general secretary of the Association of School and College Leaders, said he regretted that ministers had not responded to his pleas for them not to overcrowd the curriculum with more compulsory subjects and had instead chosen to listen to a minority.

'All special interest groups believe that their subject is the most

important,' he said. 'Regrettably, governments have a horrible habit of making more and more things compulsory and increasing the constraints on state schools.'

What they will learn
The facts of life – and when children will learn them

By age seven children will be able to:
⇨ Name the main parts of the body.
⇨ Recognise how their behaviour affects other people.
⇨ Know that families and friends should care for each other.
⇨ Understand that animals reproduce.

By 11:
⇨ Teachers should be ready to answer questions about sexual intercourse.
⇨ Children should know about the physical changes of puberty.
⇨ Recognise that puberty affects

people's emotions and how to deal with their feelings and relationships.
⇨ Judge what kind of physical contact is acceptable or unacceptable.
⇨ Resist peer pressure.
⇨ Be aware of different types of relationships.

By 16:
⇨ Understand sexual activity, human reproduction, contraception, pregnancy, sexually transmitted diseases.
⇨ Learn about relationships, that they can cause strong feelings.
⇨ Have an idea about positive and stable relationships.
⇨ Know that there are different types of relationships, including same-sex and civil partnerships.
⇨ Recognise the importance of marriage and stable relationships for bringing up children.

24 October 2008

© *Guardian Newspapers Limited 2009*

Sex education plans: too much, too young

Plans to extend sex lessons to primary schools would undermine parents and damage children's wellbeing, the Christian Institute says

In July a report by the Mental Health Foundation and Girlguiding UK concluded that 'premature sexualisation and pressure to grow up too quickly' is affecting young girls' mental health.

Last month a sexual health group, the **fpa**, launched a sex comic which asked children aged six and seven to identify correctly the vagina and testicles on a picture of a naked girl and boy.

Another sex education resource produced by Channel 4 Learning asked five-year-olds to point out the clitoris.

This week, columnist Ross Clark wrote in the *Times* that too much sex education simply gives youngsters the impression that they are expected to be engaging in early sexual activity.

Mike Judge, Head of Communications at the Christian Institute, said: 'Secondary schools already provide sex education. Extending this to primary schools is a step too far. It will undermine parents as they face the difficult job of bringing up their children.

'The best people to teach children about sex and relationships are their parents. In a culture that is obsessed with sex, schools should be one place where children are allowed to get on with life without facing pressure to deal with things they aren't ready for.'

23 October 2008

⇨ The above information is reprinted with kind permission from the Christian Institute. Visit www.christian.org.uk for more information.

© *Christian Institute*

Less glove, more love

Rachel is all for promoting condom use, but thinks sex education would be loads better if teachers and nurses actually talked about relationships too

We are bombarded with adverts explaining to us that if we want respect, we must use a condom. This is all well and good, but perhaps we might be even more worthy of respect if we didn't go around having sex with people we barely know in the first place.

'When did it become ridiculous to think that sex and love should go together?'

When I was in Year 11 the school nurse did a lesson on contraception and STIs. She said: 'Now guys, I should warn you that in Nottingham there's a lot of syphilis, so be careful! Ha ha.' Were we supposed to find this funny? It's not like it's coming after us. If we want to go around having casual, unprotected sex then yes, we may catch syphilis. But there seems to be something missing in this message. There's no suggestion with sex education that maybe it would be better to wait until you're with someone you love, or at least really like, to have sex. The message I'm

By Rachel Royles, age 17

getting is: wait until you're 16 but then you're free to go around shagging whoever you like, as long as you use a condom.

One of my friends is planning to wait until she's married to have sex. She's a Christian and believes that sex was created for marriage; she has no intention of sleeping with anyone for a long time. While this may be a very traditional and old-fashioned idea, you would think that a school nurse (who's trying to stop us catching STIs) would support her in this. However, when my friend explained that she didn't see that there was any reason for her to take condoms to a party just in case the school nurse said: 'Well, that's a nice idea, but a bit unrealistic really. It's much better for you to just carry condoms, better safe than sorry!' When did it become ridiculous to think that sex and love should go together?

Another thing that bugs me is that you can get the morning after pill before actually having sex. Apparently the Government is well aware that people are going to have casual sex so they'd rather make this pill readily available to try to stop people getting

pregnant. I really can't see how having this pill available so easily is going to discourage anyone from having unprotected sex. If two people are in a situation where they want to have sex but don't have a condom, there's less chance they're going to say: 'Damn, maybe another time' and more chance a girl will say: 'Screw it, I'll just take the pill tomorrow'. To me this seems absolutely ridiculous. Sending out the message that we shouldn't be having unprotected sex because of pregnancy and STIs while also giving out a pill which only eliminates the risk of getting pregnant seems to be contradictory.

Of course it's up to individuals to decide what they believe about sex, but I've seen nothing within advertising or sex education to suggest that having sex with someone you really trust and care about might actually be a nice idea.

Rachel, 17, is studying for her A-Levels. She's obsessed with The Mighty Boosh *and loves meeting new people and hanging out with friends.*

⇨ The above information is reprinted with kind permission from TheSite. org. Visit www.thesite.org for more information.

© *TheSite*

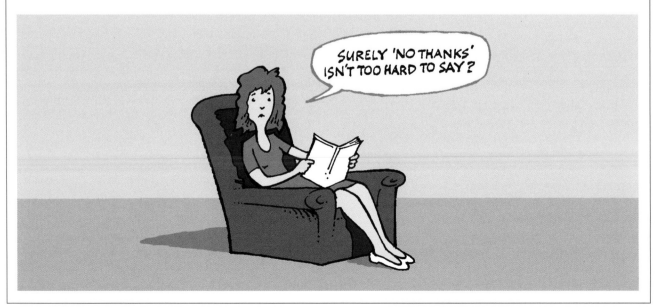

Just say 'no' to abstinence education in the UK

By Simon Blake, Chief Executive of Brook

Abstinence education is not an approach to sex and relationships education. It is worth reiterating this point, especially as the Government is reviewing what sex and relationships education is going to comprise as part of statutory PSHE – something professionals in the field cannot welcome enough!

In the UK we have signed up the UN Convention on the Rights of the Child. This gives children the right to education, health services and the right to be involved in decisions that affect them.

We have a broad consensus among young people, health, and education professionals that sex and relationships education, as defined by the Sex Education Forum, is an entitlement for all children and young people, including those with disabilities and those who are gay or lesbian.

A very small number of people in the UK persist in advocating abstinence education as a helpful approach in our efforts to reduce teenage pregnancy and promote positive sexual health. We have already seen this approach fail in the USA.

The difference between the two

Sex and relationships education is lifelong learning about sex, sexuality, emotions, relationships and sexual health. It involves acquiring information, developing skills and forming positive beliefs and values. Done well, sex and relationships education supports understanding of different views and beliefs as well as moral autonomy (Sex Education Forum 1999[1]).

Abstinence education, on the other hand, is prescriptive and offers one moral way of life, namely, 'no sex until you are in (heterosexual) marriage'.

It does not focus on the broad range of social and emotional skills required

to get the most enjoyment out of life, nor does it encourage acceptance of difference and diversity. It does not cover subjects like sexuality, STIs or birth control. Most importantly, it ignores the fact that young people are naturally curious and experimental. Young people need to know how to protect themselves from unplanned pregnancies and STIs.

Sex and relationships education is enabling whilst abstinence education is prescriptive.

The evidence

The most recent review of evidence showed that 86 per cent of the decline in teenage pregnancy in the United States was owing to improved use of contraception, with increased use of the pill and condoms. Only 14 per cent was attributed to a decline in sexual activity (Santelli et al 2007[2]).

The evidence for abstinence education, despite significant claims of success, has never been shown to have positive long-term impact on sexual health outcomes.

The moral case for sex and relationships education is strong, and so is the evidence. So, as advocates of positive education and

prevention driven by evidence and equal opportunities, let us not give abstinence education a bigger stage than it requires.

In 2001 at the launch of *Emerging Answers* (Kirby 2001), Douglas Kirby said the jury was still out on whether abstinence education was effective. In 2008 in the UK the case is closed – our energy must focus on high quality education and services, and the promotion of choice and rights. Anything less will miss the mark.

References

1 Sex Education Forum (1999) 'The Framework for Sex and Relationships Education', Sex Education Forum.
2 Santelli, J.S et al (2007) 'Explaining recent declines in adolescent pregnancy in the United States: the contribution of abstinence and improved contraceptive use'. *American Journal of Public Health*, January 2007, Vol 97. No.1

November 2008

⇨ The above information is taken from the Sexual Health IAG newsletter, November 2008, and is reprinted with kind permission from the Independent Advisory Group on Sexual Health and HIV. Visit www. dh.gov.uk for more information.

© Crown copyright

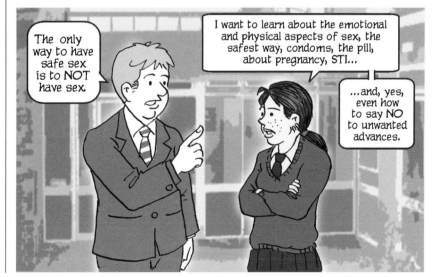

Just the jab

Schools will be at the forefront of a campaign to stop girls getting cervical cancer later in life. Carol Davis reports

Schools are the key to a new cancer vaccination programme that has the potential to save hundreds of lives. Women in this country have a 1 in 116 chance of getting cervical cancer at some point in their lives – it is the second most common cancer of women worldwide.

Health professionals are excited about the vaccine: the Department of Health says it could save around 400 lives each year. The programme, which Cancer Research UK calls 'an exciting step towards preventing cervical cancer in the UK', is being launched through primary care trusts (PCTs) from September – and virtually all of them are focusing it on schools.

Mick Brookes, general secretary of the National Association of Head Teachers, believes schools will embrace the scheme: 'If this is to the benefit of young people in preventing an unpleasant disease, then schools will welcome it, and will want to cooperate to make sure that timetabling issues are taken into account.'

The series of three jabs will be offered to year eight girls aged 12-13 from September, with a catch-up programme for older girls. The vaccine will protect against two strains of the human papilloma virus (HPV), which is spread by sexual contact and causes 70% of cervical cancer. One large-scale study from countries where the vaccine has already been introduced shows a 43% reduction in pre-cancerous changes.

The Royal Society of Health, a public health charity, wrote to all secondary school headteachers last month. 'Educational support from schools is paramount to ensuring that there is good uptake of the programme, by helping young people and their parents understand that this is an effective and necessary measure to improve public health,' the charity's chief executive, Professor Richard Parish, pointed out. The charity will publish a curriculum-support package on sexual health in July.

A Cancer Research UK study has found that three-quarters of mothers favour vaccinating their daughters against HPV. But schools have some reservations. The head of Tolworth Girls' School in Kingston-upon-Thames, Clarissa Williams, welcomes the vaccination programme but has concerns about the implications.

Women in this country have a 1 in 116 chance of getting cervical cancer at some point in the lives

---

'It does put more pressure on schools, and while we welcome anything that will protect against dangerous diseases, it perhaps needs to be balanced against other health decisions, such as the removal of the BCG vaccine for tuberculosis, or the continuing campaign against obesity,' she says. 'While health authorities quite rightly see schools as a good way to access young people *en masse*, this puts further pressure on schools' resources.'

Health professionals point out another potential issue: some parents fear the vaccination could encourage promiscuity. 'The emphasis needs to be on cancer prevention, because that is key,' says Sharon White at the School and Public Health Nurses' Association (Saphna). 'We don't want the emphasis to be on sexual health, because of the religious and ethical issues around it, although obviously it is linked to sexual health and sexual activity.'

'It is a huge public health issue, and should be treated in the same way as, say, rubella – and separated from issues around sexual health – to succeed,' agrees Kathy French, sexual health adviser at the Royal College of Nursing.

Responsible behaviour

But Williams believes that, for the vaccination programme to be truly effective, it needs to be part of a full educational programme around responsible sexual behaviour. 'It needs to be a shared responsibility with parents as part of a sensible debate about sexual health and relationship education, and I would like parents to be involved in the discussion.'

Since schools are key, how can they help to ensure that the vaccination programme saves lives? Countries that have successfully introduced such programmes have relied on a familiar leader in each school – the school nurse is the obvious choice – to work with PCTs on issues around allergies and consent.

School nurses have a vital role because of their existing relationships with schools and young people, says White: 'We should be there to answer the difficult questions of parents and carers, because we work in a school environment and community setting too.' But there are serious shortages of school nurses, according to Unite and the Community Practitioners' and Health Visitors' Association (CPHVA).

Since the programme will mean three separate jabs, observers are also concerned about girls missing a vaccination through absence. Some families will fall through the net, White believes, and the problems will be greatest in disadvantaged socio-economic groups: 'We have concerns about some of the more vulnerable children, such as looked-after children in public care, or children who are school-phobic.' She is concerned about girls with mental health issues, those with poor school attendance rates, and those who are carers themselves.

Schools will need to schedule time carefully. 'We know that this is very disruptive to education, and so schools will have to schedule so we don't disrupt the same lesson each time,' White says. Tailoring the programme to PSHE classes could help, she suggests.

Building 'herd immunity' means vaccinating a high percentage of girls, researchers have pointed out; if this fails, then boys, who carry the virus, may eventually have to be vaccinated too.

As well as timetabling the vaccination programme for year 8 girls from September, Westonbirt Independent Girls' School in Gloucestershire is setting up vaccinations for years 12 and 13 girls privately at a local hospital. 'We are pro-active about health, and we think this is marvellous,' says Susan Bath, Westonbirt's senior nursing sister. 'Some parents will be against it, but we think this is wonderful given how many women are exposed to HPV in their lives.'

Sweets afterwards

Girls can whip each other up into hysteria while queuing for a jab, but Bath believes keeping the groups small helps to defuse tension. She usually compares the process to ear-piercing, which most girls say does not hurt; she also offers sweets immediately after the vaccination.

There are many unknowns with any new vaccination programme, says Ros Godson, professional officer for school-age children's health at Unite/CPHVA. 'To make this programme work, we need to make it part of a wider remit of issues around puberty, sexual health and cancer prevention, and looking after yourself,' she says. 'It must be far wider than a stand-alone issue.'
27 May 2008
© Guardian Newspapers Limited 2009

Finger on the pulse

Jade Goody's story is more effective than any health campaign. By Max Pemberton

Jade Goody. I am aware that just the mention of her name will have some readers rolling their eyes and turning the page. But bear with me. Since leaving the Big Brother house in 2002, Jade has lived her life in the media gaze and it seems she intends to continue to do so, despite her recent diagnosis of terminal cancer. Her decision to allow camera crews to follow her through her illness has attracted much discussion and debate, with some arguing it is undignified and crass.

This tabloid favourite is no stranger to controversy and is used to polarising public opinion. But whatever you think about her, she clearly has a fan base and a significant media presence. Perhaps unwittingly, since her diagnosis she has done more to raise awareness of the importance of screening for this disease than any public health campaign.

On Internet chat sites, young women are offering support to Jade and encouraging each other to have cervical smears. They have read the interviews in which she discusses death, and seen the pitiful photographs of a bald, frail Jade. Now, everyone knows about this disease and how, if left untreated, it can be a killer.

But what she also did last week was to expose the inconsistencies in healthcare in the UK, which make a mockery of the NHS founding principle of equality. On the back of Jade's high-

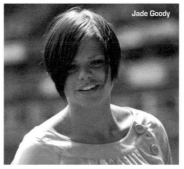
Jade Goody

profile case, the sexual health charity Marie Stopes International called on the NHS to lower the age at which women are first offered a smear test to 20. This had been the age when they first began screening until 2003 when it was raised by NHS cancer screening services to 25, after research suggested a negative effect.

This was because experts said that in their early 20s, there was evidence that women had natural changes in their cervical cells, which could be mistaken for pre-cancerous changes. This would lead to unnecessary treatment, which can lead to complications in later life, including difficulties carrying a baby to term. But on closer examination, the debate that Jade has sparked is concerned with the NHS in England only, because the rest of the UK screens at the age of 20. Since devolution within the NHS, there have been numerous examples of inconsistency and unfairness.

Prescription charges, access to medication, waiting times, hospital parking charges; the NHS is no longer consistent across the nation. In a nationalised service, there is something fundamentally wrong if such discrepancies exist. There remains debate about the appropriate age at which screening should begin, with no consensus across other European countries. But it seems ludicrous that people who are served by the same institution receive different treatment based on where they live, when the very ideological underpinning of that institution is the abolition of inequity within healthcare.

Whatever the correct age is to begin screening, young women somewhere in the UK are being let down by the devolved NHS. Either it is those in England, who should be offered it at a younger age and are therefore being exposed to an increased risk of a potentially fatal disease. Or it is those in Scotland, Wales and Northern Ireland, who are risking unnecessary, invasive treatment that can result in them miscarrying in the future.

It is the role of the NHS to evaluate the research and draw up protocol accordingly. This should have nothing to do with where you live. The NHS should treat you the same – whether you're in East Ayrshire or East Anglia. Or 'East Angular', as Jade Goody would say.
20 February 2009
© Telegraph Group Limited, London 2009

KEY FACTS

⇨ In the UK, you can legally have sex after the age of 16 (from 2 February 2009 the law in Northern Ireland changed from 17 years old to 16 years old). This applies to heterosexual sex (between a male and female), or homosexual or gay sex (between two members of the same sex). (page 1)

⇨ Around 30% of young men and women have had sex before the age of 16, so that means 70% – the majority – haven't. (page 2)

⇨ 51% of people said they would always, and 14% said they would never or rarely, use a condom with a new sexual partner. (page 3)

⇨ Frequent use of alcohol and other drugs is associated with high numbers of sexual partners and decreased likelihood of using protection. (page 3)

⇨ 34% of young people aged 14 to 17 surveyed by YouGov rated their parents/guardians as having given the most valuable advice about sex and relationships. (page 4)

⇨ In an international index measuring one-night stands, total numbers of partners and attitudes towards sex, Britain comes out ahead of America, Australia, France, Germany, Italy and the Netherlands; making the British the most promiscuous of any large western industrial nation. (page 6)

⇨ Nearly 50 children a day call ChildLine because they feel under pressure to have sex or lack basic knowledge about sexual health, relationships, pregnancy and puberty, figures have shown. (page 7)

⇨ Nearly a third of men and a quarter of women aged 16-19 had heterosexual intercourse before they were 16. (page 8)

⇨ The UK has the highest teenage birth and abortion rates in Western Europe. (page 9)

⇨ The total number of new episodes of selected STIs in men and women aged 16-19 years seen at genitourinary medicine (GUM) clinics in the UK rose from 46,856 in 2003 to 58,133 in 2007, an increase of 24 per cent. (page 9)

⇨ 87 per cent of men and 94 per cent of women aged 16-24 years knew that Chlamydia is an STI. (page 10)

⇨ A substantial proportion of teens surveyed in Scotland and England (30%) regretted their first intercourse. (page 11)

⇨ Teenage boys think there is nothing wrong with using alcohol and other tactics to pressure girls into having sex, a new study has found. (page 13)

⇨ As many as one in three 16- to 24-year-olds (32%) has had a drunken one-night stand they went on to regret, indicates a report by YouthNet. (page 13)

⇨ The Health Protection Agency has reported a 6% increase in the total number of new sexually transmitted infections (STIs) diagnosed in 2007 compared to 2006. (page 15)

⇨ There are at least 25 different sexually transmitted diseases with a range of different symptoms. These diseases may be spread through vaginal, anal and oral sex. (page 17)

⇨ In a survey of sexual attitudes and lifestyles in Great Britain, 10.8 per cent of men and 12.6 per cent of women aged 16-44 reported ever having a sexually transmitted infection. (page 20)

⇨ Just one in three adults (33%) say they always use a condom with a new partner, a time when it really is important to take precautions. Surprisingly, one in ten Brits (11%) are still too embarrassed to buy condoms – a figure that is just as high amongst older adults as it is amongst Britain's teenagers. (page 22)

⇨ Some 340 million new cases of curable sexually transmitted infections (STIs) occur every year. The figure does not include HIV or other viral STIs – including hepatitis B, genital herpes and genital warts, which are not curable. (page 23)

⇨ In 2007/08, three-quarters of women in the 16-49 age group reported using some form of contraception, with 28 per cent of women using the pill, compared with 24 per cent who relied on the male condom. (page 25)

⇨ Two-thirds of people who are at risk of contracting sexually transmitted infections have never attended a GUM clinic and said they wouldn't do so unless they were suffering from symptoms. (page 28)

⇨ Young people are more likely to use sexual health services if they can access them at schools, according to research by the University of the West of England. (page 30)

⇨ Sex education is to be made a compulsory part of the national curriculum in primary and secondary schools under government plans to cut teenage pregnancies and sexually transmitted infections. (page 34)

⇨ Women in this country have a 1 in 116 chance of getting cervical cancer at some point in their lives – it is the second most common cancer of women worldwide. (page 38)

Abstinence education

A form of sex education that advocates not having sex prior to marriage, excluding other forms of sexual health advice such as the proper use of contraception. This has become more common in the United States in the past decade, and some groups have expressed concern that the approach is gaining a following in the UK.

Age of consent

The age at which an individual can legally have sex. In the UK, the age of consent is 16 for both men and women, whether they are heterosexual, homosexual or bisexual.

Cervical cancer

Women in this country have a 1 in 116 chance of getting cervical cancer at some point in their lives, and it has recently come to the fore after the reality television star Jade Goody died of the disease. Although cervical cancer is not a sexually transmitted infection, in 70% of cases it is caused by the human papilloma virus (HPV), which is spread through sexual contact. Because of this, a new vaccination programme to inject year eight pupils against the disease has been controversial, with some people expressing concern that the vaccination will encourage reckless sexual behaviour amongst young teenagers.

Contraception

Contraception is used during sexual intercourse to prevent pregnancy. Barrier methods such as condoms are also effective in preventing sexually transmitted infections. The most common types of contraception are condoms and 'the pill' (the combined or mini contraceptive pill). Emergency contraception such as the 'morning-after pill' can also be used for a limited period after sex to prevent a pregnancy, but will have no effect on sexually transmitted infections.

GUM clinic

GUM is an abbreviation for genitourinary medicine. GUM clinics specialise in diagnosing and treating sexually transmitted infections. They can also offer advice about STI prevention and contraception methods. Services are always offered confidentially.

One-night stand

A one-off sexual encounter with someone who you are not in a long-term relationship with, and with whom you may not be well acquainted. It is very risky to have a one-night stand with someone if you have no knowledge of their sexual history, and especially so if a condom is not used.

Promiscuity

Having a high numbers of sexual partners. This can be risky as the greater the number of sexual partners, the greater the risk of catching a sexually transmitted infection.

Sex and Relationships Education (SRE)

Sex and Relationships Education takes place in schools; its purpose is to help young people acquire information and form attitudes about sex, sexual identity, relationships and intimacy, so that they can make informed decisions about their own sexual activities and avoid unwanted outcomes such as unplanned pregnancy or catching sexually transmitted infections. The Government announced in October 2008 that SRE was to be made a compulsory part of the national curriculum in primary and secondary schools in an effort to tackle teenage pregnancy and the spread of sexually transmitted infections.

STIs

Sexually transmitted infections. These can also be called STDs (sexually transmitted diseases), but the term 'infection' is sometimes preferred over 'disease' as some STIs (such as Chlamydia) can be symptomless. The term 'VD' (venereal disease) may also still be used as another name for STIs. Common curable STIs are gonorrhea, syphilis and Chlamydia. Some 340 million new cases of curable STIs occur every year. Viral STIs such as genital warts, herpes and HIV are treatable but cannot be cured.

INDEX

Additional Resources

Other Issues *titles*
If you are interested in researching further some of the issues raised in *Sexual Health,* you may like to read the following titles in the **Issues** series:

⇨ Vol. 171 *Abortion – Rights and Ethics* (ISBN 978 1 86168 485 1)

⇨ Vol. 174 *Selling Sex* (ISBN 978 1 86168 488 2)

⇨ Vol. 164 *The AIDS Crisis* (ISBN 978 1 86168 468 4)

⇨ Vol. 153 *Sexual Orientation and Society* (ISBN 978 1 86168 440 0)

⇨ Vol. 143 *Problem Drinking* (ISBN 978 1 86168 409 7)

⇨ Vol. 133 *Teen Pregnancy and Lone Parents* (ISBN 978 1 86168 379 3)

⇨ Vol. 123 *Young People and Health* (ISBN 978 1 86168 362 5)

For more information about these titles, visit our website at www.independence.co.uk/publicationslist

Useful organisations
You may find the websites of the following organisations useful for further research:

⇨ **AVERT:** www.avert.org

⇨ **Brook:** www.brook.org.uk

⇨ **Centre for Public Health, Liverpool John Moores**

University: www.cph.org.uk

⇨ **ChildLine:** www.childline.org.uk

⇨ **Children First for Health:** www.childrenfirst.nhs.uk

⇨ **Christian Institute:** www.christian.org.uk

⇨ **fpa:** www.fpa.org.uk

⇨ **Guttmacher Institute:** www.guttmacher.org

⇨ **Health Protection Agency:** www.hpa.org.uk

⇨ **Independent Advisory Group on Sexual Health and HIV:** www.dh.gov.uk

⇨ **Lloyds Pharmacy:** www.lloydspharmacy.com

⇨ **Medical Foundation for AIDS & Sexual Health:** www.medfash.org.uk

⇨ **NSPCC:** www.nspcc.org.uk

⇨ **Office for National Statistics:** www.statistics.gov.uk

⇨ **Seduction Labs:** www.seductionlabs.org

⇨ **Sex Education Forum:** www.ncb.org.uk/sef

⇨ **TheSite:** www.thesite.org

⇨ **United Nations Population Fund:** www.unfpa.org

⇨ **YouthNet:** www.youthnet.org

ACKNOWLEDGEMENTS

The publisher is grateful for permission to reproduce the following material.

While every care has been taken to trace and acknowledge copyright, the publisher tenders its apology for any accidental infringement or where copyright has proved untraceable. The publisher would be pleased to come to a suitable arrangement in any such case with the rightful owner.

Chapter One: Sex Matters

Sex, © NSPCC, *Sex and relationships*, © Brook, *Sexual health in 2008*, © Medical Foundation for AIDS & Sexual Health, *Sex myths*, © TheSite, *Britain 'most promiscuous Western nation'*, © Seduction Labs, *Nearly 50 calls a day to ChildLine about sex*, © NSPCC, *Teenagers: sexual health and behaviour*, © **fpa**, *Teens, sex and the law*, © AVERT, *Teens positive about first sexual experience*, © Guttmacher Institute, *Under pressure*, © Christian Institute, *One young person in three has had one-night stand*, © YouthNet, *Sex and substance abuse*, © Centre for Public Health, Liverpool John Moores University, *Young people and STIs*, © Health Protection Agency, *Sexually transmitted diseases and symptoms*, © AVERT, *Sexually transmitted infections – statistics*, © **fpa**, *Brits turns a blind eye to STIs*, © Mintel.

Chapter Two: Improving Sexual Health

Breaking the cycle of STIs, © United Nations Population Fund (UNFPA), *Methods of protection*, © Cambridge University Students' Union, *Pill still the most popular form of birth control*, © Crown copyright is reproduced with the permission of Her Majesty's Stationery Office, *Pitfalls of condom use*, © Cambridge University Students' Union, *STI testing*, © Crown copyright is reproduced with the permission of Her Majesty's Stationery Office, *'Nice girls' refuse to get checked for STIs*, © Lloyds Pharmacy, *Benefits of school-based clinics*, © National Children's Bureau, *School clinics could reduce pregnancy and infection*, © University of the West of England, *Sex education that works*, © AVERT, *Where do baby rabbits come from?*, © Guardian Newspapers Ltd 2009, *Sex education plans: too much, too young*, © Christian Institute, *Less glove, more love*, © TheSite, *Just say 'no' to abstinence education in the UK*, © Crown copyright is reproduced with the permission of Her Majesty's Stationery Office, *Just the jab*, © Guardian Newspapers Ltd 2009, *Finger on the pulse*, © Telegraph Group Ltd, London 2009.

Photographs

Stock Xchng: pages 2 (Heather Haislet); 15 (Jonathan Fain); 18 (Lotus Head); 26 (Sebastian Schaeffer); 33 (tim & annette).
Wikimedia Commons: page 39 (Keira76).

Illustrations

Pages 3, 13: Bev Aisbett; pages 5, 11, 23, 36: Don Hatcher; pages 7, 16, 28, 37: Angelo Madrid; pages 8, 21, 27, 30: Simon Kneebone.

And with thanks to the team: Mary Chapman, Sandra Dennis, Claire Owen and Jan Sunderland.

Lisa Firth
Cambridge
May, 2009